The Cancer Olympics

ROBIN MCGEE

Produced by:

FriesenPress

Suite 300 – 852 Fort Street
Victoria, BC, Canada V8W 1H8

www.friesenpress.com

Distributed to the trade by The Ingram Book Company

To my parents, Robert and Janette McGee,
for their example of courage, sense, and humour.

This is a true story based on actual events. Although some individuals have been given obvious pseudonyms, real names have been used with permission.

1

I AM HOLDING A PHOTOGRAPH OF MY TUMOUR. IT WAS TAKEN over a week ago, the day of the colonoscopy. It is swollen and distended, pink skin stretched over the bulging malignancy. Almost entirely circumferential, only a tiny amount of normal tissue holds out against the freakish masses that surround it. It is bleeding vigorously, growing so fast that it is bursting its own blood vessels.

I am aswim with shock and grief. And another feeling—anger.

I stare down at it and it stares back like a baleful eye.

I think, *how did I get here?*

....

My story begins simply enough. I was raised in Ontario, the sixth of seven children. We lived in Ottawa, where my father was a senior civil servant, and my mother stayed home to look after such a large brood. An imaginative, daydreaming creature that was always reading, I grew up happily. Through having to earn my own way through university, I developed habits of hard work and self-reliance that tempered my creative and curious nature.

My ancestry was Scots and Irish, giving me an odd mixture of miserliness and sentimental passion. This character led to choosing a career that would pay well enough, while still allowing me to do something both noble and moral. Child psychology seemed a good fit. My undergraduate degree was a combined honours in English and psychology, because I could not get away from my love of books despite the need for a common-sense career.

I did well in university and earned sufficient scholarships to pay my way through. Slugging through a seemingly interminable PhD in clinical child psychology, I met my husband on a blind date. We bonded while quizzing each other about Beatles song lyrics, and I knew that I had met my match.

Andrew was a native of Nova Scotia. Work had taken him from his home province, and he pined for it. He woke up each morning thinking about how far away he was from the ocean. When I finally graduated, we moved to the beautiful Annapolis Valley (known in Nova Scotia as simply "The Valley")—a verdant, pastoral place. I was pregnant when we arrived, and our cherished son Austin was born that same year.

I went to work as the only child psychologist at the regional hospital. Eleven years and many initiatives later, child psychology had grown in the district. When an opportunity came up to join the regional school board, I jumped at the chance despite a significant pay cut. My new job required me to provide consultation to over 40 schools regarding children and youth. Between my work in health and education, I knew many of the doctors, nurses, lawyers, police, teachers, and principals in the professional system, in addition to neighbours and friends throughout the length and breadth of the Valley.

My cancer story began on 26 June 2008. I remember that date, a Thursday, especially clearly as I was working with the hospital's autism diagnostic team that day. The following Sunday night, I was to fly to Scotland on vacation with my mother and two of my sisters. We were planning to celebrate my mother's 80th birthday in the land of her parents' origin. We would also be celebrating her being free of colon cancer after a decade.

Earlier that week I had felt the stirrings of a urinary tract infection. Being prone to those, I certainly did not want to head off to Scotland with such a problem. My family doctor would not prescribe antibiotics for a UTI without all the relevant urine testing done through her office. I remembered that she once told me that if

I was really in need, I could take the Ciproflaxin that she had once prescribed in case of bowel trouble for a previous trip to Mexico. Hoping to head off the infection before it took root, I took the Cipro for two days while simultaneously going through the urine testing she required. At last convinced, she prescribed an antibiotic I had never had before—Noroxin. I switched to it promptly.

On 26 June 2008, I saw blood in my stool for the first time. Understandably disturbed, I called the doctor's office but could only book an appointment for 14 July, the day after I returned from Scotland. *This is not good,* I thought, queasy. *Maybe this is bad. Really bad.*

I shook those thoughts from my head. *Nonsense.* I was a fit, active non-smoker in my 40s. Careful eating and vigorous exercise were my daily habits. Happy in my work and family life, I had no mental health struggles. *You are healthy,* I reassured myself. *This is nothing.*

But the bleeding continued throughout my Scotland trip. It continued after the antibiotic was finished. I quelled my anxieties by reflecting that I was to see my doctor as soon as I got back home.

The day after I returned, I hurried to my doctor's office, but my own family doctor was away. Instead, I met with someone doing a locum at that practice. I shall call this person Doctor Number One.

Doctor Number One was warm and reassuring. She told me that the bleeding was probably due to the side effects of the Ciprofloxacin—that the bowel-specific antibiotic had likely disturbed the flora of my intestine, and the bleeding was a result of that disturbance. She recorded in the Electronic Medical Record (EMR) that the digital rectal exam was normal. She did not order any blood work, but instead ordered a stool sample test to check for parasites and *Collustrum Difficile.* The latter is often described as a "superbug"—a bacterial infection signalled by diarrhea and flu-like symptoms. Although I never had either of these indicators, a fact that she documented in her EMR notes ("No diarrhea"), the *C. Difficile* test was ordered anyway. She did not refer for endoscopy, despite documenting in the EMR that the blood was mixed in the stool. I told her about my immediate family history of colorectal cancer twice during our appointment, but she did not document it. She did not book a return appointment.

Dr. Number One had recently moved from another province, and she was not aware of testing standards for *C. Difficile*. Laboratory standards as early as 1996 required that that any sample submitted be liquid stool, not formed stool. So when I took my sample in that same day, the lab rejected it as unfit and cancelled the test. I never heard about this cancellation. Thinking that "no news was good news," my feelings of concern diminished. After all, Dr. One's hypothesis of an antibiotic reaction made sense to me. The bleeding stopped, as Dr. Number One guessed that it would, after a few more weeks. That cessation seemed to be the reassurance I needed.

But months later, in October, the bleeding suddenly resumed. This time, it seemed worse. Also, the bleeding was accompanied by an odd symptom—I was passing bloody sheets of skin. These sheets of skin were small, about the size of a dollar coin. They started off as translucent and pink, but within a few weeks, they had become like red, floating rags. Disturbed once more, I went to see my regular family doctor, whom I shall call Doctor Number Two. Doctor Number Two had been my family physician for 15 years, ever since my arrival in Nova Scotia. She was also a colleague I knew through my professional work; on occasion, we had patients in common that required conferencing.

Dr. Number Two seemed annoyed with me as I described my symptoms and Dr. One's ideas. She complained that I had not submitted a stool sample for the *C. Difficile* test because the lab report said "no specimen was received in plain container." I protested that I had indeed submitted a formed stool sample, but Dr. Two said she would need to order it again. I told her about the bloody skin, which she documented in her EMR notes ("blood in stool, and passing 'bloody tissue'"). I reminded her that I had an immediate family history of colon cancer, which she also documented. She did a digital exam, which was normal, and she ordered some bloodwork. I understood her to say that she would consider a referral to a specialist once the *C. Difficile* test came back. She also announced that her practice would be closing in about six weeks.

As I got up to leave, Doctor Number Two stood also. Realizing that I may never see her again, I asked what her plans were. She replied that she might take up a locum in Halifax. We looked at each other awkwardly for a moment. Ought I to hug her? Ought I to thank her for her years of doctoring?

Strangely, an inexplicable sensation of coldness came over me. I hung back awkwardly, wished her well tersely, and left, perplexed over my sudden attack of shyness and aloofness. I do not know if the shiver I experienced that day was a premonition of what was to come. If my life was the *Titanic*, Dr. Two was about to become my own personal iceberg.

After I left her office that October day, Doctor Number Two wrote a consultation request letter to a local general surgeon. Her letter said: "Thank you for seeing this most pleasant 47-year-old woman, who has had episodic bright red bleeding per rectum since June of 2008." Dr. Two had recorded many indices of very serious bowel pathology in her EMR notes, but she left all that material out of her referral letter. She said nothing about the bloody mucosal tissue, my immediate family history of colorectal cancer, my previous bowel history, or even her own exam results. Despite the risk of future miscommunication, her letter did not mention that her practice was closing. The bloodwork came back showing a positive result for C. Reactive Protein, an index of inflammation and a potential cancer marker. She did not forward that result to the specialist either.

I will never know why she withheld such critical information from that referral letter. Whatever the reason, her lightweight letter was another step in a series of cumulative failures that were to bring about my doom.

Who could I approach to be our new family doctor? My husband and son had requested a male this time. I considered a man I shall call Doctor Number Three. He had been in the same practice office as Doctor Number Two: this could mean that he would share in the EMR system she had used. File and information transfer would be facilitated, I reasoned. I knew Doctor Number Three from years of collegiality with shared patients. One day in November, I called him about a mutual patient and added in my request to become his patient. A week later, his secretary called saying he was willing to take me on. I would, she said, need to accept that I would wait on average three weeks before getting an appointment. After all, Doctor Number Two had just quit, along with two other physicians in that collective practice. Thousands of citizens were now without a family physician. I was lucky to get one at all.

Dr. Number Two's practice closed officially on December 5th. On December 9th, Dr. Number Two's receptionist called me to say that the lab had rejected the second stool sample for *C. Difficile*, as the sample was not watery.

"Where does that leave me?" I asked, bewildered.

The secretary's response was final and exasperated: "You are on your own with that," she said.

What could I do now? I would have to find a way to resubmit the *C. Difficile* test on my own. There is a district health authority laboratory in the building where I work, so I went there that December day to ask for advice. The assistant introduced me to the laboratory's consulting physician, and I explained my situation to her. She told me that both of my previous samples would have been cancelled because only liquid stool is acceptable for *C. Difficile* testing. She also said that both Doctors One and Two had been misguided in ordering the *C. Difficile* test for me, as it was only appropriate for those with a history of diarrhea and flu-like symptoms. The main concern, she said, was to determine if my bleeding came from higher up in the digestive system. She told me the fecal occult blood test (FOBT) was the appropriate test; she gave me a requisition for one along with careful instructions meant to maximize its specificity. That same day, I called my new family doctor and was given an appointment in early January 2009. I followed through on the FOBT in order to have the results ready in time. These results were, of course, positive.

I regarded Doctor Number Three as a sincere and friendly man. It felt somewhat odd to me to see him as a physician when we had related so often in the past as colleagues. Nevertheless, I told him all about my symptoms. I told him that I was passing bloody epithelial tissue. I was relieved that he nodded in agreement when I told him that the lab doctor had said the *C. Difficile* issue was a red herring. I told him about my immediate family history of colorectal cancer. He did not examine me. After listening, he said unequivocally that what I needed was a colonoscopy—that a scope was the definitive test for my issues, and that a scope required a specialist. Dr. Three emphatically promised that he would seek and arrange such a scope for me: he would call the specialist, a woman I shall call Dr. Number Four, and find out how long it would take to get me in. Expect to wait a long time, he warned.

He explained that there was nothing else he could do for me apart from ordering bloodwork to rule out celiac disease. Reassuringly, he told me that my symptom was likely nothing significant. "Sometimes," he said, "intestinal walls get thin in places— it is like you are having the bowel equivalent of a nose bleed." I left Dr. Three's office profoundly relieved because I had finally found a physician who would get help for me.

More fool me.

When Doctor Number Three saw from the electronic records that Doctor Number Two had already made a specialist referral, he decided to take no action. He never noticed the inadequacies of Doctor Two's referral letter. Even though the first two doctors had described my symptoms as lasting months, and despite the degree of detail I had given him, he summarized my symptoms in his EMR note as "three episodes of bright red bleeding lasting days." When my bloodwork came back a few days later ruling out celiac disease, he took no action. He did not forward my positive FOBT results to the specialist. Doctor Three's receptionist made an entry in his electronic records saying that a follow-up call to determine the wait for endoscopy to the specialist had been completed. But it had not been completed, and never was. So in the end, Doctor Number Three did nothing at all.

In the rural area where we all practiced, professional circles are small. For years, I had seen Doctor Two and Three socially as well as professionally; I had been on a first-name basis with them both. In addition to all the times we talked as colleagues, we attended the same parties and social events. Dr. Three and I had children in the same local theatre productions. When I had won a professional practice award in 2005, the two of them sent me flowers. I thought we had a congenial relationship: it simply never occurred to me that they would give me short shrift. Trusting them, I went along with my daily life.

The months went by. I waited for the specialist office to contact me, not alarmed at the delay as I had been warned there would be a wait. But the symptoms continued.

The first Friday in July, I was troubled by how much worse the bleeding seemed. It seemed to me heavier—a tablespoon instead of a teaspoon—and more unusual. I called Dr. Three's office. When the receptionist answered the phone, I identified myself and told her that I had seen Dr. Number Three for rectal bleeding in January, and that he had referred me to general surgeon Doctor Number Four. I told her that my symptoms were worsening, and that I had heard nothing from Dr. Four's office. Could she check to see if the referral had been sent? She checked her computer and assured me that the referral had been sent and received.

"Are you still having the bleeding?" she asked.

"Yes," I replied, "much more."

She made a supportive tsking sound and told me my best bet was to call the specialist's office and gave me the phone number. That was the end of our call. Although this receptionist was supposed to judge the clinical relevance of incoming calls and record significant ones in their electronic system, she did not make an entry for my call. Even though we had discussed my worsening situation twice during our conversation, she did not tell Dr. Three about it.

Upon hanging up from Doctor Three's office, I immediately called Doctor Four's office. When the receptionist answered the phone, I identified myself and told her that I had seen Dr. Three for rectal bleeding in January, and that he had referred me to Dr. Four. I said that my symptoms were worsening, and since I had not heard anything, I wanted to check that my referral had been received. She checked her computer and told me that yes, the referral had been received, but the wait for a scope in our region was 18 months. When I expressed my surprise and concern at such a wait, she replied that Dr. Four was very busy, and that she had access to the endoscopy equipment only every two weeks. I asked whether I might be better off to seek a consult in Halifax. She replied that the wait in the Halifax region and elsewhere in the province was "even worse." She confirmed that if I left Dr. Four's queue, I would have to wait another 18 months in someone else's queue. Discouraged, I said, "It seems I have no choice but to wait." She replied authoritatively that yes, I would have to wait because the problem was due to lack of resources. She told me that I could call her back in six months, and an appointment might be considered then. Defeated by this information, I ended the call.

After I hung up, I considered my options. What could I do? Should I go to the Emergency Room? I had always believed that ERs should be reserved for true emergencies. My symptoms were troubling, but not disabling; besides, three doctors had given me such benign explanations for them. Also, I knew that colonoscopies take a full day's bowel preparation in advance—this did not seem like something an ER would undertake.

Should I call back Dr. Number Three and ask that a scope be done out of province? Such a demand seemed drastic and overreactive, given the assurances three doctors had given me. I knew from my own work how difficult it is to get out-of-province care. Dr. Three had been emphatic with me that there was nothing else he could do for me: that a scope was the only procedure that should be done, and that a specialist had to do it. I had already seen him to expedite the referral. Surely he would have communicated to the surgeon the full history. If he had been unable to persuade her, then my wait must be the result of a valid triage decision. Besides, the three doctors I had seen seemed to think my symptoms were the result of an insult done to my intestines from an antibiotic—nothing serious. So I waited.

I trusted them. I did not know not to.

Unbeknowst to me, Dr. Four had long ago abdicated her responsibility to triage her own surgical cases to her receptionist, a secretary with no medical training. I had a previous file at Dr. Four's office, having seen her for an anal fissure 12 years previous. My immediate family history of cancer was clearly described in that file. But Dr. Four's secretary did not pull existing charts on patients when making her triage decisions. When my referral came in, she put it at the very bottom of the pile. Because Dr. Four had developed the belief that all her colleagues had wait times as long as hers, she instructed her secretary to tell patients who called that the 18-month wait was a provincial norm.

By Christmas 2009, my symptoms had escalated to pain. I had my first episode of severe constipation. I called Dr. Four's office again to report my intensifying symptoms and insisted on an appointment. This time, the secretary granted me a consult time with Dr. Four in February 2010.

It was with a feeling of relief and consummation that I walked into the office of Dr. Number Four. Dr. Four joked affably with me about Blackberry phones being "crackberries" as she called me in from the waiting room.

She pulled out my thin file. "You are here for the same thing I saw you for 12 years ago, right?" she said.

I felt a prickle of alarm. "No, that was just an anal fissure," I said. "This is something much worse."

She shrugged and looked at the consult note in front of her. "But this just says you are bleeding from the bottom end," she said.

That's all it says? I wondered, mystified. What about all the detail I had given Doctors One, Two, and Three? As she turned the page on her desk, I could see that she had a very brief paragraph in front of her, no more than a few sentences. I began to feel uneasy. She was not taking me seriously; indeed, she seemed determined to take a light view of my case.

"So," she said, "what makes you feel that this is something more?"

As I related my history, she would interrupt with presumptive questions. "You only have pain when you poop, right?"

I tried to clarify. "No, Dr. Four. I have pain all the time. It is a continuous, throbbing ache." She wrote "no pain" into her notes.

I told her all my symptoms: the by-now copious bleeding, the constipation and undue frequency, the bloody discharge mixed with mucus. She was unimpressed. Dr. Four interrupted my history frequently with questions to which she seemed to have already determined the answer.

"You only bleed once every few months, right?"

"No, Doctor Four, I bleed every day."

"But every few months, it is worse, right?"

"There are days when the bleeding is worse, yes."

"You have not had any bleeding in a few weeks, right?"

"No, Doctor Four. I had very heavy bleeding with a lot of stool frequency just this past weekend."

She had me on the examination table for the digital exam. There was dark red blood on her examining glove. "There is a hemorrhoid there," she said laconically. "Nothing to write home about."

When I was back in the chair in front of her desk, she tapped the bloodwork results lying on her desk. "Your January bloodwork was fine, and you have no abdominal symptoms," she said briskly, "so I think that this is a mild case of inflammatory bowel disease, probably just a proctitis, a mild inflammation of the rectum."

"I understood that I was referred for a colonoscopy," I said. I was uncertain if I should feel relieved or uneasy by her apparent certainty.

She considered. When she finally said, "I suppose we should do one anyway to be sure of what we are looking at," I sighed with relief.

As I was crossing the threshold of her door, I was struck by the realization that I did not have bloodwork in January 2010—she had based her consult on bloodwork from *January 2009—more than a year before!* I turned to knock on her door, which had closed behind me. The secretary saw this and called me over. I told her, worried, that Doctor Number Four had mistakenly used old bloodwork when forming her opinion.

The secretary called up the bloodwork results up on her own computer. "Yes," she said, "that was from January of 2009, but it does not matter. She has scheduled you for a scope about three months from now. Today I will give you a requisition for bloodwork for you to do about six weeks before the scope. That is routine."

"But you will tell her, right?" I asked anxiously.

"I will let her know. Now here are the forms you need to complete."

That same day, Doctor Four wrote a consult letter to Dr. Three. It was filled with inaccuracies and omissions. She noted but was not concerned by my family history. "Family history was positive for colorectal neoplasia in her mother when she was 69," she wrote, "but there are no other family members with colorectal neoplasia." Her consultation letter expressed her doubt that I could have cancer: "I would have expected it would have progressed to being more symptomatic, if it was a neoplastic lesion." Dark red blood is another alarm symptom for cancer, but Doctor Four wrote, "a digital rectal examination was normal although there was a small amount of maroon coloured blood on the examining glove." She went on to express how mild my symptoms were, basing her impression on my "January bloodwork." Her letter stated: "Robin had a CBC done *in January of this year* which showed a hemoglobin of 125...her ESR was only 4. C Reactive Protein was negative." She never noticed that the bloodwork she was referring to was from over a year *previous*—the results ordered by Doctor Number Three, thirteen months earlier.

I reassured myself that in three months I would finally have the long-awaited scope. *So I have inflammatory bowel disease*, I thought. *That makes sense.* The internet confirmed that rectal bleeding and a feeling of rectal fullness are symptoms of IBD. When I had consulted the internet previously, it had said that rectal bleeding accompanied by anemia and weight loss is indicative of cancer. *Good thing I do not have those symptoms.*

Open to learning things about my presumed condition, I went to a learning day for Crohn's disease and ulcerative colitis. I watched the videos and heard the speakers. The questions from the audience about ostomies, internal pouches, and steroids were piteous. The audience was reassured that the new immunosuppressant drugs came with only a four percent increase in the risk for colorectal cancer. *These poor people*, I thought. *I am lucky that my case is not so severe.* I was the sickest and most endangered person in that audience, and I did not know it.

On 6 May 2010, I went in for the colonoscopy—22 months after I had first reported my symptoms to family doctors, and 18 months since Dr. Two had referred me for specialist investigation.

I lay down on the table, flanked by two nurses. Doctor Number Four held up the scope end. "You are just the same as when I saw you in February, right?" she asked, although it was more of a pronouncement than a question.

"No, Doctor Four," I said. "I am much worse." The pain and dysfunction had escalated so much in recent months that it had become noticeable to my friends and family.

The colonoscopy really hurt. The nurses had to hold me down.

"There is a growth there," said Doctor Four when it was over. "I will set up a time for you in the next week or two."

Through my sedated fog, I heard the word "growth."

That night and the following days, I experienced extensive bleeding and constipation. *A growth.* I knew what that must mean.

That week after the scope was among the worst I had ever experienced. I moved through my workplace like a hunted animal, avoiding the eyes of friends and co-workers. I knew something, but I could not tell it.

My friend Barbara, a breast cancer survivor, read the note of anxiety in my emails to her. "It is not cancer," she reassured me over the phone, "until they say it is."

But it was.

Eight days after the colonoscopy, Doctor Four took me and my husband Andrew into my office. "You have colorectal cancer," she said, slapping a photograph from the scope down in front of us. It showed a nearly circumferential malignancy, bulging and bleeding.

"You will need radiation, chemotherapy, and surgery," said Doctor Four. "You will need a permanent colostomy. The treatments will put you into premature menopause. I will be your surgeon, but the rest of the treatment you have to get through the Cancer Care Centre in Halifax. I will order a CT scan and an MRI to tell us what stage it is. I am guessing, looking at this photograph, that you will be in a very advanced stage. Because it is Friday today, the referral will get looked at sometime next week."

When we asked why I had not been triaged for a colonoscopy appropriately, Dr. Four rolled her eyes. "The wait is long because there are no resources here," she said.

"What about Halifax?" Andrew asked.

"The wait in Halifax is *even longer*," she said emphatically.

"But why was Robin not a priority even here?" he persisted.

She shrugged. "Because she was under 50 years old," she said simply. "And besides, for every one like her, there are hundreds who just have hemorrhoids."

"This must be very tough news for you to have to deliver," I said, wondering what it would like for her.

"And I have three other people to give this news to this morning," she said impatiently, indicating the door.

....

I look down at the photograph again, trying to swallow down the despair and anxiety, but fighting a backwash of revulsion and rage.

I am staggered and sickened to learn that Dr. Four and her receptionist had misinformed me about the 18-month wait for a scope in the province. It was not, and had *never* been, commonplace *anywhere* in Nova Scotia for symptomatic patients to wait that long for endoscopy. Within days of my diagnosis, I meet colleagues, some in their 20s, who had been scoped within weeks of their symptom onset by other Valley doctors. *Dr. Four* maintained such a lengthy wait time as a norm within her practice, but no other specialists did. I am stunned to learn that in 2004 the Canadian Association of Gastroenterologists had specified a recommended wait time for endoscopy for rectal bleeding of only eight weeks. *Eight weeks.*

Like a hazy photograph sharpening into focus, my perception of what had gone wrong develops into realization. My eyes are opened, and the enormity of the flaws in my medical care is heartbreakingly revealed. Each doctor had been superficial, each one careless. Each one expected some other doctor to take responsibility for my care—so in the end, none of them did. Each one had failed to communicate effectively with me and with each other. Not one of the four physicians ever even mentioned cancer to me as a possible explanation for my symptoms. If even one of the doctors had described cancer as the possible differential diagnosis, I would have been even more aggressive in my search for appropriate assessment—I would have known to fight harder at the delays and roadblocks I encountered. Now, I can never get that time back again. All unaware, I had been in a "perfect storm" of medical mismanagement.

There is no point in shock or regret. *Not even God can change the past*.

I am going to need everything I have in me to endure the radiation, chemotherapies, and surgeries I will require in order not to leave my only child motherless.

2

I PUT DOWN THE PHOTOGRAPH OF MY TUMOUR.

I must make the phone calls, I force myself to think. I pick up the receiver. *So it begins.*

My first call is to my supervisor at the Annapolis Valley Regional School Board. Cindy is expecting me at a meeting with resource teachers in a few hours.

She is shocked. I ramble as I talk to her, naively saying that I will be in to make the meeting. She interrupts me, supportive but firm—I must cease my direct service work in schools effective immediately. From this moment on, she tells me, I will work only from home. She assures me she will make all the necessary arrangements with Human Resources.

And next my parents. My father and mother are stunned. After the first exclamations of pain, they find words. My father announces with confidence that he knows I can beat cancer. He tells me that I have made him proud in the past, and that recovery will be another such accomplishment. They remind me that my mother had survived her stage IIB colon cancer 12 years ago with flying colours.

I feel sickened to compose it: an email to my six brothers and sisters.

And then another, to my friends.

As I write, I hear the familiar clunk of my son's book bag landing on the floor in the front hall. He is home from school.

We call him into the kitchen. We tell him to sit down.

I cannot get my head around this. Words come out of my mouth and I point at pictures in the brochure Dr. Four gave us, but I cannot focus on what I am saying. *The next years of his life will be terrible. I am sentencing him to...what? I cannot get my head around this.*

Austin is speechless. He reaches out towards me to clutch me and hugs me closer. His face is bewildered. I press my forehead to his, an act of affection we have used since he was small. I am too choked up to speak.

This is the cruellest part, I think. *Nothing is worse than the prospect of bereaving your child. Nothing.*

....

Ron Hurst is my father–in–law. After he retired from Irving Oil, he and his wife Christine followed their dream. They sailed their 32-foot yacht *Rhumb Runner* down to the Caribbean, where they both found work in the British Virgin Islands for a yacht company. He kept the fleet of vessels for hire in repair, whereas she worked the business end of addressing the needs of the guests.

When Ron was 60, he developed a persistent sore throat. Their health insurance plan allowed them private health care in the US. Ron went to the prestigious Mayo clinic in Florida. He was given the diagnosis: squamous cell esophageal cancer. A clumsy doctor scoped his throat without the usual protections and forced the cancer cells into his stomach. It spread, eventually moving to his lungs and lymph. The brutal treatment regimen involved radiation, feeding tubes, multiple surgeries, and chemotherapy. Ron faced it—indeed, he outfaced it. Months of devastating treatment, of vomiting through a damaged stomach through a raw radiated throat, of harrowing disfigurements (they removed every one of his teeth)—but he beat it. He beat it all. He left that clinic declared cancer-free.

Ron returned to his work in the Caribbean. For another nine years, he lived well. The radiation had damaged his capacity to make saliva, so he had to wash his food down with beer. Visitors were agog at how fit he seemed: he could stand in powerboats that crashed against the waves at high speed, he could spend hours focused on mechanical repairs, and he could work and play in the Caribbean sun seeming no worse for wear.

But in the fall of 2009, his sore throat returned. No longer able to access private health care, he had wisely arranged for residential status in Newfoundland. He was seen at the St. Clare's Mercy Hospital. Yes, the cancer was back. He could not have more radiation—surgery was his only option. We will remove your throat, they told him, and replace it with a tube made from intestine. You will lose your voice, they added. "I love you," were the last words he said to his wife when they wheeled him away to surgery.

Ron astonished the doctors and nurses with his remarkable healing powers. He was up and vital within a week.

But three weeks later, the new throat would not "take." Perplexed, the doctors were determined to repeat the surgery and give him another new throat, this time using skin from his leg. So Ron underwent a second surgery.

Again, Ron's apparent recovery amazed and impressed all the staff. Again, he was up and vital within days.

Three weeks later, they told him that they found another tumour, growing behind his new throat. Another surgery was not an option. Perhaps he would be willing to undergo chemotherapy? Ron refused—he wrote that he would rather die than go through what he had endured 10 years ago. No, they assured him, this drug was different. It was gentler. It was his last and best chance.

Ron tried the new chemotherapy. Within minutes of taking it, he had an intensely negative reaction. Later analyses revealed that he had an extreme intolerance to it. The oncologist that spoke to Andrew about it was in tears. There was nothing left, nothing more they could do.

So Ron went home, back to his beloved islands, knowing he would die there in a matter of weeks. He sent out an appeal to all his children: come see me one last time. He did not want us to come to a funeral after his death. He wanted us to come to the islands, to spend a week in a beautiful villa loaned by a friend. So we all booked our tickets—Andrew and I and our son Austin. So did Holly, Andrew's sister, and her husband and two newly adopted daughters. Ron's daughter Mandy had been estranged from him for over 20 years, but she and her husband Stewart will go too.

Ron's oncologist told us that July will be too late. He has only weeks left. If we are to see him before the end, we must go *now*.

But I have just been diagnosed with cancer.

Now we have anguishing choices to make. *What will we do about Ron?* Dreadful questions press against my apprehension. *Am I safe to travel? Should Andrew go to the islands without me?* How desperate and unsupportive that seems to me. I cannot bear to deprive him of the chance to say goodbye to his father, but I fear starting cancer treatments without him. Andrew would certainly refuse to leave me when I will be so vulnerable.

But still my head is swimming in shock. *How can this be true?* I am a fit, highly active professional in my 40s. I have never smoked. I have eaten a careful healthy diet since childhood. I worked out nearly every day. I had played women's 7-Aside Soccer for 14 years. In the five years I had worked for the school board, I had only taken a few sick days in total. And yet, I must absorb the realization that I am in the grip of a lethal disease, and that my life is about to take a radical and sudden departure.

....

Days later, I arrive at Valley Regional Hospital for the MRI. They told me on the phone that the CT scan will have to wait for the following week. Saying goodbye to Ron seems increasingly impossible.

The MRI technician has a familiar face. She tells me that she knows me from some help I had arranged for her stepdaughter some 10 years before. Trembling, I explain to her our dilemma about Ron—I need to know whether I could go to see him before his death. How can I leave the country if I have to stay for the CT scan that would determine my staging? And for what that staging would reveal?

Inside, the MRI is dark and close, like a warm cocoon. I hear my own breathing. Despite its banging sounds, I find myself falling asleep, the exhaustion of the past few days overwhelming me at last. Over the headphones, the technician keeps calling to me to rouse me.

When I emerge, she leads me to another room. A large glass of viscous liquid is waiting for me.

"I had a little talk with my friends in CT," she says, "and it makes sense to me that you get your Cat Scan today as well. After all, you already have an IV in, right? So why not?" She offers me the glass of Gastrografin. *God bless you*, I murmur in my heart. *Thanks to you, maybe I can go to the islands after all.* I wonder what happens to those who do not have friends on the inside of health care.

Other technicians operate the CT scan. I try to explain the situation regarding Ron. I point out that the CT requisition has the words "URGENT" in capitals on the top of the page. I ask them if they will communicate the urgent status to the radiologist.

"No we won't," one responds, shaking her head. "If we tell him that your case is considered urgent, he will deliberately put it at the bottom of the pile. He does not like being told what to do."

Underneath my bewilderment, I feel a great gaping, a falling away. *Can a radiologist really be that passive-aggressive? Even if he was, why would hospital staff tell a cancer patient about it?* I see, as if from a precipice, a bird's-eye view of cancer care. Doctors do only what they want to do when they want to do it. Cancer care is a hopeless map of conflicting personalities, motivations, and whims. Patients have no control. *We are at their mercy*, I think. *There are no standards.*

....

Dr. Jan Hux is a specialist in internal medicine from Ontario. She is also a recent survivor of a very harrowing experience with breast cancer, not back at work yet. A mutual friend has asked her to call me.

Jan spends hours with me on the phone: explaining, clarifying, reassuring, and normalizing my terror.

When I eventually obtain copies of the CT and MRI results, I read them to her over the phone.

"The MRI says 'a 4-5 cm irregularly thickened segment of rectum originating at about 8-10 cm from the anal verge...with evidence of a 1.8 cm lobulated focal region of extension beyond the rectal wall with probable associated demoplastic reaction making the lesion a T3 tumour stage'," I read to her. "'There are a few small scattered adjacent perirectal lymph nodes which are mildly enlarged and a small moderately enlarged right internal iliac chain lymph node highly suspicious for early nodal metastatic disease.' The CT scan report also identifies lymph node involvement, including a '1.1 cm right internal iliac lymph node.' What does all that mean?"

Jan pauses before she answers.

"You need to think of this as good news," she says carefully. "Usually, circumferential tumours the size and shape of yours mean that the cancer has spread to many organs. I expected to hear it was all through your pelvis. I know it is strange to hear this, but you must consider yourself very lucky. There is a chance your cancer might be *treatable*."

I blink. Until this moment, I had not grasped that it might not be treatable.

Jan listens empathically to my torturous doctor story. I share my anguish over their omissions and delays. How can I stop this kind of outcome from happening to other patients? How can I address the wrongs that were done, particularly by Dr. Number Four? How do you complain about someone who will have you under a knife? I tell Jan that my inquiries in the medical community have revealed that Dr. Number Four has not done regular GI surgery in years.

"You need to find another surgeon," Jan says emphatically. "Research is clear that survival from any cancer, but particularly rectal cancer, depends on the skill of the surgeon. You want to find someone who does rectal cancer surgeries *every week*. You want someone who really knows how to spare muscles and nerves during surgery, so that you can have the best possible function afterwards. Besides, when it comes to cancer, you have to be able to trust your treatment team. If you cannot trust Dr. Four, you *must* find another surgeon."

She offers to email various colleagues to find out who would be the best surgeon in Nova Scotia. When the many replies come in, she forwards to me the responses of various national and international experts. Although many names are mentioned, one man is repeatedly identified as "the best hands in the business": Dr. Bernie McIntyre.

I will find him, I promise myself.

....

Andrew and I are in the examination room of Doctor Three. On the office wall, Dr. Three has tacked up hundreds of pictures of himself with his children. His computer screen shows him as the star of a rotating cascade of pictures: dropping a hockey puck between two focused boys, cradling a newborn baby, dandling a grinning toddler. Dr. Three's young son grins happily from the photos. I reflect that when my son was that age, he was just as sweet, just as fragile, just as trusting. I swallow painfully, reflecting that Dr. Three's beautiful children get to grow up with both their parents, but my innocent son may not.

I hold in my hands a typewritten summary of my assessment experiences. Dr. Three enters, anxiety tugging at his features. He settles into his office chair, his eyes darting, and he clears his throat. He starts off with a practiced "doctor" voice.

"The biopsy says you have moderately differentiated adenocarcinoma," he says. "This is the typical colorectal cancer. And while I know the images show a lesion on your liver, it is probably a benign cyst. Many people have them."

I hand him the document I have written, summarizing in one page my assessment history. "I want you to read this," I say.

After he has read it, he lowers it slowly. His hands are shaking.

"When I learned of your diagnosis," he says weakly, "I went home and cried. I...I never did the follow up I promised, Robin." He adds feebly, "I thought Dr. Two had referred you, so I didn't call Dr.

Four. I made a note in the electronic medical record for my secretary to call Dr. Four to see how long it would take to get your scope, and somehow it got signed off as completed. But no one called her. It was just a computer mistake, maybe just a couple of wrong keystrokes...I am...I am sorry."

Dr. Three reaches over and tries to grab my hand. "Maybe it would not have mattered what I did or did not do," he adds breathlessly, "because Dr. Four might have refused me just the same way she refused you. When resources are scarce, some specialists dig in. And if I had ordered other tests, say a barium enema, that probably would have missed your cancer and made the situation worse, delaying the scope even more..."

I am too stunned to speak.

"You did nothing for me after I saw you, asking for help?" I say, realization dawning. "Nothing at all?"

Dr. Three shrugs and looks down. "I meant to."

I point to the narrative, still clutched in his hand. "I want this entered into my medical file, to be on the permanent record."

This strikes Dr. Three as funny. "Permanent record? Permanent record!" he scoffs. "You have been with the school system too long." He laughs aloud at his joke.

I do not laugh. "I am pretty well known in both health and education, Doctor Three," I say. "Soon the whole region will hear about me, and about this."

I watch the colour drain from his face.

"If you want to atone for what you did," I say, "you must get me a new surgeon. I would like to see Dr. Bernie McIntyre."

"Atone?" He looks bewildered. "Atone?"

"We want a new surgeon, and we want you to tell Doctor Four that I will not work with her. And to tell Doctors One and Two about what happened here. I will send this document to you as a pdf, and I want you to send it to them."

Dr. Three looks shellshocked. *What does it feel like to have seriously harmed a patient through failure to act?* I wonder. *It must feel truly terrible.* Beneath my own despair, I pity him. I hug him before

I leave his office. *I bet*, I think prophetically, *that there is more to this story.*

We emerge from his office. Above the regional hospital, we see dozens of crows circling in the summer sky.

"Remember a few years back when the sky would be black with crows above the hospital?" Andrew asks.

"The sounds of their screams was overwhelming," I recall. "It used to hit you like a wall as soon as you left the building."

"What is the word for a large group of crows?"

I watch the black birds alight on the roof of the hospital.

"Murder," I answer, swallowing hard. "It's called a murder of crows."

....

I struggle to understand my diagnosis. All I have is a booklet, *Colorectal Cancer and You*, put out by the Colorectal Cancer Association of Canada. It teaches me that most colorectal cancer evolves from the adrenal glands within the colon or rectum. It begins as a benign polyp on the innermost layer of the intestine—the part closest to the food. A polyp can develop into a benign tumour called an adenoma. Over time, an adenoma can progress to become malignant, at which time it is called adenocarcinoma. In this sequence, the tumour can grow through some or all of the tissue layers that make up the intestine. It can spread beyond it, into the lymph nodes, and then to other distant nodes or organs. Survival is highly conditional upon detection and treatment at the early stages. Once it has spread to distant organs, it is considered incurable. After lung cancer, colorectal cancer is the most common form of cancer and the leading cause of cancer-related death.

I am dizzy and distraught to read the section on prevention and early detection. Colorectal cancer is similar to skin cancer in its preventability. As polyps grow, they bleed. Even microscopic amounts of blood can be detected using fecal occult blood tests, like the FOBT I had done. When such bleeding is found, it should trigger prompt endoscopy. Using such tests, most provinces and states have moved to universal screening programs for average-risk individuals over the age of 50. People with an immediate family history are considered to be high risk, as are those with a history of inflammatory bowel disease. High-risk individuals must have more intensive surveillance, typically by colonoscopy. The most common symptoms are blood in the stool, changes in bowel habit, iron-deficient anemia, and weight loss. Blood mixed with stool, particularly in the absence of hemorrhoids or fissures, is considered an "alarm symptom" for colorectal cancer; it merits endoscopy, ideally within 60 days.

I want to cry. From the day I walked in to a family doctor's office with semi-urgent symptoms to the day of my endoscopy, my wait was not 60 days—but *661 days*.

The prevention booklet breaks my heart. It reads: "If you have any of these symptoms, talk to your family doctor."

....

The Nova Scotia Cancer Centre is located at the Queen Elizabeth II Health Sciences Centre, on the second floor of an old hospital called the Dickson Building.

We enter through the big double doors that separate cancer patients from all others. We take our number and sit down in the central waiting room. It is appointed with folk art, quilts, and pictures dedicated in memoriam. Volunteers hand us cookies as we take our seat.

I look around. I am by far the youngest person in the waiting room. *Is that good?*

When our turn comes, we are beckoned into an examination room by a young nurse in a white lab coat. She introduces herself as Cara, our radiation oncology nurse. When she asks me how my symptoms developed, I hand over my assessment history document. In my mind, I have entitled it "The Perfect Storm of Medical Mismanagement."

"I cannot keep repeating this terrible story," I say. "We are asking all our treatment providers to read it."

"Oh my God," she says under her breath as she reads. When we add that Andrew's father Ron is dying, and we want to be with him before the end, she rises to her feet. The paper is trembling in her hand.

"I am going to find you your medical oncologist right now," she says firmly. "I will find out a date for you. And I will give this story to your radiation oncologist to read."

Our radiation oncologist enters. Dr. Gaurav Bahl is new to the Cancer Centre. A dignified young man with soulful brown eyes and a cultured accent, he shakes our hands and draws his chair up close to us. For over 90 minutes, he listens to us and responds to our questions. We ask him the same questions repeatedly, and he answers each one patiently as if it were the first time. His pager goes off. He checks it, silences it, and returns to his respectful listening. *He understands that he is our first encounter with the cancer care system,* I think. *He understands how fearful, desperate, and bewildered we are.*

Dr. Bahl describes how treatment will unfold for me: there will be three main components. The first step will be chemoradiation—28 days of radiation, concurrent with chemotherapy. The intention is to shrink the tumour as much as possible before surgery. I will need to come to the Cancer Centre for the radiation every day except weekends and holidays. He will design the radiation course and will follow up with me once a week. The second step is surgery. The third and final step will be months of additional chemotherapy. Before I can begin treatment, I must do two things: I must be marked with tattoos to help target the radiation beams, and I must see a medical oncologist—a specialist in chemotherapy.

"Can we go and see Ron before his death?" we plead. "If we do that, will it delay my treatment?"

"You may as well go," Dr. Bahl reassures us. "It will take a few weeks for you to get on the machines anyway. You will need to see the medical oncologist before we can start, and I think the next available appointment will be after you return."

Cara comes back in the room. She confirms that the next available medical oncology appointment is two weeks away, with a Dr. Mark Dorreen.

We go home and pack for the islands.

3

EACH OF US LEAVING FOR THAT ISLAND HAS A STORY. I HAVE cancer, and I am going to see a man struggle in the end stages of the disease I have just been told I have.

Holly, Andrew's sister, and her husband, Steve, have only months before adopted two little girls from Family and Children's Services. J is 9-years-old, and H is one year younger. The girls have a painful and troubled history, including a previous failed adoption. For most of their little lives, they have been in foster care. These youngsters have never been in a cab before, let alone an airplane or a foreign country. Holly and Steve are understandably anxious about their adjustment, and about how they might respond to the emotionality of the week before us.

Andrew's other sister Mandy has been estranged from her father for over 20 years. Ron has never even met Stewart, her husband of 15 years. Mandy has only one week to rediscover her father, and he her, before his death—and he is no longer able to speak.

Andrew has spent the past 10 months supporting Ron through the final stages of his illness. He had been there when they told Ron there was no longer any hope. He is exhausted and demoralized, lost between despair and the burden of my need.

"If this were a movie," Steve remarks, "no one would believe it. We would say: 'who writes this stuff?'"

The plane ride is uneventful. We arrive in the dark close heat of the tropic night. The air is sweetly scented with bougainvillea and the distant ocean. I go straight to bed, troubled with physical and emotional pain. My mind darkens as I retreat into brooding...*Why did this happen to me? What had gone wrong with all those doctors? How could they possibly have been so collectively negligent?* I torture myself, wondering if I could have anticipated it. I ruminate about Dr. Two, who had been my family doctor for 16 years. I had always considered her to be so professional and knowledgeable, if sometimes sceptical. *Had she dismissed my description of the bloody mucosal tissue as mere fancy on my part? In her hurry to get out of her practice, was she rushed and forgetful? Had I hurt her feelings by my less-than-warm departure, and was the superficial job she did a result? Or was she just a fallible human being who had made a series of thoughtless mistakes?* These questions spill around in my mind like laundry in a dryer. Dr. Two has not contacted me since learning of my diagnosis, which hurts me. *I will never know why she acted as she did.*

But despair leaks around those thoughts like sewage from a rusty pipe. *The past does not matter.* What matters now is crisis, my crisis—whether I can live, whether I must leave my husband and child, my work, and my identity...just as Ron was losing these things now. *Can I endure these treatments?* I have heard about two colorectal cancer patients who each lost 60 pounds during treatment. *Sixty pounds!?* I had weight to lose, but not 60 pounds. The stories I hear of the pain and suffering endured by cancer patients freezes my blood. I hear of those who vomit so forcefully that they lose their teeth. I hear of bleeding radiation burns. I hear of desperate, prolonged, and agonizing deaths.

The next morning, we meet Ron and his wife Christine. Ron is very, very thin. *He is dying of starvation*, my mind registers. He is grey, all grey, and his blue eyes are rimmed with white. The bolus of his tumour pushes visibly out of his throat, below the tracheotomy.

He hugs us. He nods and gestures to convey us out to the dock where a borrowed powerboat is waiting.

Leverick Bay BVI is breathtaking. Mountains lush with verdant vegetation rise steeply from the harbour. Colourful sailboats line the marina, with many more at restful anchor. On the waterfront, a cheerful bar is playing salsa music.

Christine, Ron's wife, tells us that our villa is well up the mountainside. When we arrive alongside, the men unload the suitcases to the quayside. Ron grabs a pull lever on one of the suitcases and starts up the steep hill, dragging it behind him.

I do not see the accident. Andrew, Steve, and Stewart are hauling the suitcases up the mountain when they hear the crack. Ron has fallen, face first, into the rough pavement. His face and jaw are covered with blood. When they raise him to his feet, they see that his teeth have cut right through his cheek.

They assist him up the hill to the villa. Ron lies down on the couch, his mute countenance alive with shame and disappointment. He covers his face with his hands.

He lies there silently as we unload the rest of the gear. Eventually, the pain and despair drive him to his bed.

The villa is a beautiful open-concept dwelling. The walls are windows onto a breathtaking vista of purple clouds against an azure sky and a sparkling ocean. The tropical winds usher in the heat-driven scent of flowers. A veranda, complete with several inviting hammocks and chairs, encircles the villa. Looking down, we see a panorama of gorgeous gardens, spilling down the cliffside. The heat is close and sensual. Everywhere there is the perfumed softness of the tropics, ineffably lovely.

In my heart, and in the hearts of the others, there is a heavy, unreasoning dread. The contrast between the exotic beauty and our deepening grief is stunning and surreal.

....

We awake each morning to the ecstatic cries of birds. Each day, we gaze out on heart-stopping loveliness and exuberant growth. Each morning, we attempt to walk up the hill for exercise before the sun becomes too hot. Each afternoon, we listen to the sounds of the girls joyously shouting as they splash in the pool. And each night, we lie staring at the ceiling, our minds and bodies gaunt with tension and sorrow.

Mandy spends hours sitting beside Ron, holding his hand. He sometimes rallies sufficiently to show her pictures on his laptop. For the most part, he lies on the couch, sleeping or sometimes reading. Occasionally, he writes notes to communicate. Many of these convey his growing despair and depression. "It is terrible to lose control of your body," he writes in one. "It is eating me."

How can I answer this? I wonder. *How close am I to understanding his terror firsthand?*

In the afternoons, I lie in the hammock and listen to my ipod. Before leaving for the islands, I had downloaded several cancer-specific visualization mp3s from *Health Journeys*, my favourite internet source for guided imagery audio. In my psychology practice, I had often recommended their imagery mp3s to people struggling with insomnia, depression, and anxiety. Their oncology offerings prove to be tender, warm, social, exalting, soothing, and even humorous. One mp3, spoken by the mellifluous Psychologist Emmet Miller, describes radiation as a big barbeque—cancer cells are sizzled on the grill by the radiation beams, and ravenous white blood cells swarm to feast upon them.

As I listen, I gaze out at the azure bay, stunned at the prospect of losing my life and forfeiting forever the beauty of this world. I am to be parted from the splendour of nature, just as surely as I am to be parted from Ron, and we will both go down into the dark.

One morning I wake up bleeding. I am startled, afraid. *Wait, this can't be. I just had my period two weeks before.* In my 40 years of menstruating, I had never had two periods close together. Under stress, I typically stop having my period. *And this is unusually heavy.* A grey and grim idea grasps my heart and crushes it. *Could the cancer have penetrated my reproductive system?* The bleeding gets heavier with each passing day.

My fears are escalated by the obscurity and remoteness of my surroundings relative to the medical world. The nearest medical facility is several islands away. The phones, the internet, and the electricity keep going down. *Who can I reach for help?*

After hours of frustrating effort, I learn the emergency contact number for the Nova Scotia Cancer Centre. I reach the radiation oncologist on call. I describe where I am and what is happening. Andrew is sitting beside me, anxiously clutching my hand.

My breath runs out as my words die. "I am so scared," I finish helplessly.

The voice of the radiation oncologist is calm. "This is unlikely to be a cancerous invasion to your uterus," she says, "if it was not evident on your recent MRI. Instead, I think you are under incredible stress. I will review your MRI with Dr. Bahl tomorrow and have him call you. Worst comes to worst, you can get yourself packed—I mean packed internally—to stop the bleeding and fly home."

The phone lines come back up the next day. When we are able to get through to Dr. Bahl, he is reassuring.

"We looked at your MRI again," he pacifies me, "and we believe that the bleeding you are having is not related to the cancer. We will start your treatment once you are home. No need to worry."

I receive another call. I am standing on the wraparound porch, facing the gorgeous view of the Caribbean Bay, with the cellphone to my ear. A warm alto voice announces that she is Leslie Snide, the secretary to Dr. Bernie McIntyre. She has tracked me down to this remote island to tell me that Dr. McIntyre has agreed to take over my case, and that he will see me next week. I want to sink to my knees in relief.

That night, my hemorrhaging stops. But Ron's begins.

We are sitting around the supper table. Thankfully, the girls have gone to bed. We are apprehensive with anticipatory grief. Mandy must leave tomorrow.

Sounds of drums and partying boom from the harbour. We can hear the whoops in the distance and the brazen cacophony of drunken laughter and salsa music. Tonight is a special night in Leverick Bay; each year on this night, the wealthy of Puerto Rico come over in their speedboats for a noisy and vibrant celebration.

Ron staggers into the room. His face and the front of his shirt are covered with blood.

He gestures wildly at us. Blood is burbling out his mouth.

Chris springs to her feet. Seizing the phone, she calls the medivac service. She repeats aloud what she is being told: a powerboat has been dispatched from another nearby island. It will arrive at the government wharf near the main resort dockside. It will take him to the hospital on another island. He must go down to the dockside immediately.

The jeep is hastily readied. Blanched with fear and distress, Ron's children gather beside it. Each family member reaches out to him to hug him or touch him as he climbs inside.

He could die tonight. Ron rolls his hands to gesture the driver to speed on, a bloody handkerchief pressed to his mouth. His eyes are alive with fear.

We run through the perfumed air, rushing down the hillside towards the dock, our hearts pounding.

Fireworks explode overhead as we arrive panting at the government wharf. We hear singing and shouting amidst the ecstatic music, as Ron collapses onto a bench at the end of the dock. Our anxiety is overwhelming. The carnival atmosphere clashes in bizarre juxtaposition to our primitive terror, as if we were in a surreal scene from *Apocalypse Now.*

Two inebriated doctors break off from their convivial party and wander loosely over to us. Breathless, Andrew and Chris explain Ron's situation.

Swaying where he stands, one of the doctors offers to look Ron over.

"Open up," he says, slurring his words slightly. "Looks stable to me...I think the bleeding has stopped for now. Sometimes these tumours just bleed."

A powerboat swivels up to the wharf. Two medics jump out. The first quickly assesses Ron as the other talks to the drunk doctor.

"Sir," says the examining medic to Ron. "Your vitals are stable now. However, we think you need to come with us to the hospital just to be sure."

Ron shakes his head piteously, gesturing for paper. He writes: "That is not how I will spend my last night with Mandy."

The family expostulates with him, but he continues to shake his head. He stands up on shaky legs and walks away, starting down the wharf to the hillside. He is going back to the villa.

The medics shrug. "It is his decision," they say. We follow Ron as he starts back up the mountainside.

We lie awake all night, wondering if Ron will survive until morning.

In the morning, Mandy departs. We all of us, Ron included, walk her down to the wharf where the water taxi will take her away from her father. She openly weeps, her head hanging and her shoulders shaking as she sobs. And I weep too: for her, and for my own child, who may soon have to say goodbye to a parent forever.

....

Little J approaches me with a book in her hands. "Will you read us a story?" she asks tentatively. "*Harry Potter?*"

I read to J and H with animation and gusto. I notice that both girls are looking at me earnestly, watching my face with wide eyes. *They know*, I guess. *Their parents finally told them about my diagnosis.* I am relieved.

"Your Mom had cancer," J interrupts.

"Yes she did," I reply.

"But she is still alive."

"Yes, she is."

J considers this information. She puts her head to one side, her little brows knit.

"Can she talk?" she asks.

....

It is the day of our departure. We are waiting on the tarmac outside the island airport.

Ron hugs each of his children and grandchildren. They are struggling with emotion, too overcome to speak.

Ron comes up to me last. His white-rimmed eyes are expressive. He points at my chest, raises his fist, and shakes it.

"You fight," I interpret for him through my tears. "If anyone," I choke, "has been a model of fighting, it has been you."

Ron and Chris hold hands as they walk away from us, towards the sea. He does not look back. Just before he crosses over the horizon, he lifts his arm in a salute. We will never see him again.

4

BEING DIAGNOSED WITH CANCER IS LIKE BEING CLUBBED ON the head and thrown into a deep mud pit. You are stunned and disoriented, and you stagger in a place you cannot get out of, no matter how much you claw at the walls. And the monster is coming.

I am devastated by this diagnosis; although in retrospect, when I reflect on my symptoms, it all falls into place like an evil jigsaw. Like the optical illusion in which a vase becomes two faces, I suddenly see my past shift into a new and hideous focus: ignorant benignity becomes cruel laughing malignancy.

I watch people in the street, going about their lives. They seem so separate from me, so safe, as if I am watching them from behind glass. *How can I get back on the other side?* I scrabble for books or internet information that can guide me. But no information can change the fact that the alien is inside me—growing, always growing. I think of the images of the cancer-stricken I have seen on television: emaciated sufferers who look like the famished inmates of a concentration camp. I remember once hearing that those who die of cancer most often die of starvation. *Is that my fate?*

"Cancer" is the most feared word in the English language. Confronted by it, every bodily instinct for fight or flight is aroused. Only flight is not an option. Between each action of my day— between picking up a fork and putting it down again—I have a million thoughts that dart back and forth between acceptance and anger and fear like an animal in a cage.

And suddenly there is death. My death. Something so easy to ponder in the abstract, but so crushing and appalling when it looms right before me. The knowledge that death by cancer is not just any death freezes my soul. I read an oncology paper in which the writer opens with "Death by peritoneal cancer is the cruellest death imaginable." *More cruel than what?* I react in despair. *Being burned to death? Tortured to death?* Although I am not afraid to cross over into death, I am afraid of great suffering. And, more agonizing even than the thought of relentless and hopeless pain, is the incalculable grief of leaving my child.

Friends sometimes say things that restore me to hope. When I express to Thea my sorrow at the prospect that I will not get to see my child grow up, she replies flatly, "You will not die. Your purpose in this life is not accomplished yet."

The certainty in her voice arrests me. I feel full of purpose still: for my family and my work. But can my commitment to life protect me?

My friend Kym comes over to help me garden. She has recently lost a close friend to ovarian cancer. Diagnosis to death in her friend's case had been only weeks.

"But you are different," she says to me. "Your energy and perspective on life are just different. Your spirit will ensure that you survive—I am certain of it."

Others respond with calmness. "I have ESP," one says. "And I know, just *know*, that you will be fine in the end." Their confidence is comforting, but I find myself hanging on to their faith like a frightened child clings to her mother.

I do not waste any time blaming myself or God for my cancer. As a psychologist well acquainted with human suffering, I know that bad things happen to good people. After the misery of years of futile treatment for secondary infertility, I know that I am not special. I know that we live on a poisoned planet and in a fallen creation. The genetic mutations of cancer blight animals and even plants: why would I be exempt? I could brood endlessly on the toxins I have been exposed to. Was it the pesticide-laden apple I had eaten three years ago? Was it the "sick building" I had worked in for years? I recognize all those thoughts as both useless and burdensome, with the potential to drive me even deeper into the mud pit mire.

I am often asked if being a psychologist makes coping with the anxiety of cancer any easier for me. Yes, I answer, but only in the daytime.

I am tormented by vivid nightmares. In one, I am clinging to the outside of a train that is rocketing down a precipitous landscape. In another, I stand inside a barn on the other side of an enormous stall door. Behind the door, I can hear the snuffing and pawing of a powerful bull I am condemned to fight. Through the door, I can sense that it is supernaturally large. In another, my mother and I are in a house. My mother is knitting in a chair in the bedroom, unaware that near her on the white bed an immense coal-black python lies coiling and uncoiling. It is gathering its potent lethality and animal strength to kill us. I seize my mother and we both escape outside the house. Gasping, I wake up in alarm.

To overcome the chilling vestiges of these nightmare visions of the evil and power of cancer, I repeatedly watch youtube videos of a mongoose killing a cobra. I want to supplant those terrifying images with those that prove that even the mightiest snake can be defeated by the small and the brave.

But even nights without nightmares are sleepless. There is too much to take in, too much to integrate, too much to plan, too much to dread.

My pain is increasing. My stool has become as thin as a pencil. The bleeding is copious.

....

We are in the waiting room of the Cancer Centre, awaiting our first visit with the medical oncologist.

We are called over by a nurse. She introduces herself as Lynn. She tells us that she had worked in palliative care for years before coming over to medical oncology. A warm embracing personality, Lynn offers encouragement as she takes my history.

"You look 10 years younger than you really are," she reassures me. "Maybe you will sail through this."

When she hears that Dr. McIntyre will be my surgeon, she is delighted. "Dr. McIntyre!" she exclaims. "That man is so gifted, I would let him operate on my child's brain tomorrow!"

She reassures us that Dr. Dorreen, with whom we will meet shortly, is a similar kind of specialist. "He is head of the department here," she says, "and has been an oncologist for 30 years. And like Dr. McIntrye, his technical competence in oncology is extraordinary. You are in the best hands there are for your kind of cancer."

I hand her my Perfect Storm document. As she reads it, her face betrays her shock and distaste. "I will put this on your file," she says with a shudder. "And I will ensure that Dr. Dorreen reads it before he sees you. You need the best of medical care from now on. No more mistakes." She departs to brief him. We wait.

When Dr. Dorreen comes in, we stand to shake his hand. He is an avuncular bear of a man, with the comportment of a senator and the resonant British voice of a Shakespearean actor. When we ask if he has read the Perfect Storm document, he acknowledges that he read "the essay" Lynn had given him. He examines me, carefully palpating my liver.

He listens intently to my description of my worsening symptoms. I hand him the photograph of the tumour taken the day of the scope.

My practiced psychologist's eye detects the shocked recoil that crosses his face before he can conceal it.

"It is really bleeding vigorously," he says, his features shifting into an expression of worry, his thick brows contracted with concern. "And your stools are getting thinner...When did they tell you the radiation can start? You need treatment as soon as possible."

He reviews my treatment path. He explains to us that rectal cancer tumours, unlike colon cancer tumours, are in a small confined space, surrounded by bone and other organs. Surgical outcomes and survival chances are improved by shrinking the tumour as much as possible before the resection surgery. Thus, my treatment must begin with combined chemotherapy and radiation. The intention is to make the tumour more susceptible to the impact of radiation—to make the cancer cells weak and staggering before radiation delivers the knockout punch. To do this, I must undergo infusion of the chemotherapy Fluorouracil, also known as 5FU, through continuous infusion. A special catheter called a PICC line will be inserted into a large vein in my arm and fed right up to the main vein near my heart where the blood flows quickly. The 5FU will be attached to the PICC line by means of a bottle I must wear 24 hours a day for the six weeks of radiation. Acting as a pump, my own heart will circulate the chemotherapy. He adds that the major chemotherapy I will receive after the surgery will be of a different nature, and that we will wait until after the surgery to discuss it.

After Dr. Dorreen leaves, Lynn comes back in. She has checked the schedules. I can start in two weeks.

"Dr. Dorreen read your doctor story," she confides. "He thinks you could not have had cancer for two years."

"What else could it have been," I ask, "if not cancer?"

"Maybe an adenoma, or precancerous bleeding polyp. He said anyone with your kind of cancer would most assuredly be dead if they had it for two years. You certainly have a very, very large tumour. No one can understand how you are even standing."

Lynn pauses. "Sometimes," she muses, "I think that things happen for a reason. The reason for what happened to you may not be clear yet. But something important might come out of your story. I have a feeling about that."

But I had symptoms for two years, I wonder. *Why am I still alive?*

I am about to find out.

5

News of my condition has spread through our region. Within days, the phone is ringing off the hook, with friends, family, and colleagues in a state of bewilderment. In my incarnations in the Annapolis Valley, I have been a hospital psychologist, a teacher at the local university, a school board psychologist, and a soccer player. People from all those walks of life come forward—with prayers, with encouragement, with offers of help. Gifts, flowers, and food show up at my door. Within days, I have received over 60 personal cards from well-wishers. Messages and emails pour in. I am contacted personally by just about everyone I know, or had ever known.

One of the surreal aspects of a cancer diagnosis is that you get to hear your own eulogy before your death. Friends and family come forward to tell you what you have meant to them, remembering what you have done to help and support them. They recall fond adventures or work accomplished together. I am touched and stunned to realize how connected I am, and how significant I have been to many—and they to me.

My colleague Stephanie lost her brother to cancer the year before. Only 32, he was a gifted endurance athlete. The doctors dismissed his ever-increasing thinness as a result of his running. When he finally underwent the right investigations, he was discovered to have a metastatic stomach cancer that was well past the point of intervention. When he died, he left a wife and three small children—the youngest only eight months old. His extended family rallied to support him and his family throughout his ordeal. Stephanie passes on to me a resource they had found valuable: an online support site entitled *Lotsa Helping Hands*.

While his wife Carole was dying of ovarian cancer, businessman Barry Katz tried valiantly to care for her needs, raise his two daughters, manage the household, and maintain his work. The family was planning the Bat Mitzvah for his youngest daughter Julia when the oncologist told them they ought to reschedule it sooner—that his wife would not live to see it otherwise. Amidst his personal devastation, Mr. Katz strove to rearrange the event: the caterers, the DJ, the temple service. Friends and family came forward to help him. Mr. Katz used an office whiteboard to document and manage all the tasks with which he needed help. When the day came, Carole was able to look on from her wheelchair as her daughter read from the Torah and gave a sermon on its meaning: she spoke of love, of family, of community, and of "lots of helping hands." Carole died six days later.

Barry Katz wanted his family's struggle to count for something. He wanted to develop a free online service that would help other families overwhelmed by a crisis. He named it after something his daughter had talked about in her Bat Mitzvah sermon: www.lotsahelpinghands.com. Based on the white board he had used during his own crisis, the site allows volunteers to offer practical help. The stressed family can specify the kind of help that is needed (e.g., meals, rides, childcare), and volunteers can sign up for specific tasks. The site also allows for simultaneous communication of announcements using push email. Lotsa Helping Hands also allows for community members to express well wishes and access media such as documents, photos, or videos. It is a simple way for overstressed families to reach out to relatives, friends, and neighbours for help in getting through their day-to-day lives. Since its inception, it has helped over 25,000 families worldwide through tough times that no one should have to face alone.

Lotsa Helping Hands also combines flexibility with security. To create an online community, one can invite people to join via email and judge the acceptability of email applicants. Only those approved by the coordinators can join the community. Logging in even once meant that future announcements arrived by ordinary email, so members did not have to continually check a website. If someone wished to make a statement for the entire community to read, they could post it on the website under Well Wishes or a Message Board. Alternatively, if he or she wanted to reply to an announcement email privately, they simply used return email. Their response would come to me alone, not to the entire community. Creating a community is simple, instantaneous, and free.

My friend Thea Burton comes over to help me set up the website. Together, we navigate to the Lotsa Helping Hands homepage.

Thea bends over the computer. "Here is the place for the name. What should we call it?"

My kitchen table is covered with get-well cards. I walk over to it and pick up one from those that crowd the table.

I turn back to Thea with the card in my hand. "Let's use what Beth Robinson has written here," I say. "Let's call it 'Robin's Cancer Olympics.'"

I post my first announcement:

WELCOME
posted to LHH by Robin McGee, Friday, June 4, 2010, 3:30 PM

Welcome to our "Robin's Cancer Olympics" Lotsa Helping Hands Website!

Robin has entered the radiation, chemotherapy, and surgical events. With her friends, family, colleagues, and other teammates cheering her on, it is widely predicted that she will pull off a gold medal victory in each event!

This site is where you can stay tuned for updates on her training and condition. Also, for those who are willing to help out Robin and her family, there is a calendar that allows helpers to register for helpful things. There is a comment section for well-wishers, for those that want to express encouragement.

Within days, friends and family respond to the Olympic metaphor:

We are with you Robin
posted by Joelle C at Sunday, June 6, 2010, 7:12 PM

Got the original post and we are now walking with you on your Olympic path!

Go for the Gold!
posted by Krista L at Monday, June 7, 2010, 9:06 PM

Hey Robin,

Looking forward to seeing you on the podium..."I Believe."

Friends from TMP
posted by David C at Wednesday, June 9, 2010, 5:51 PM

Hi Robin...this is a great site!! The staff at TMP school has also joined you on your march to the gold medal. Your passion for what you do everyday at school and your amazing sense of humour has obviously not changed. Good luck with your treatments...please get well soon...

David and staff

The Olympic Analogy
posted by Pam S at Wednesday, June 9, 2010, 11:09 AM

Hey Rawb:

I love this analogy as it clearly involves all the factors necessary—training (both physical and mental), competing, and finally, winning!! Yes we can!! I love our walks—it feels like therapy for ME!! XXOO

Warm Regards and Energy from GES

posted by Corena B at Thursday, June 10, 2010, 4:52 PM

Hi Robin,

As our staff is learning of your news, their sad faces quickly change to "What can we do?" We are sending you all of our warmth and energy through this email to fill your reserve. We will chart your progress and sing "O Canada" as you achieve victory! Love ya, from all of us from GE School.

My hugs and love to you! This will be a challenge to your spirit, but baby you have it in you! Thanks for allowing us to share this with you and to be on your "bench!"

Enjoy the Day :)

posted by Tara S at Saturday, June 12, 2010, 8:32 AM

Just wanted to pass along some advice from my five-year-old son, who was going to shout it up to your window yesterday—to win the Olympics, you have to try your best, be a good sport, and have fun. So I think you've already got your strategy down because I can't imagine you any other way (I would have trouble with the good sport thing myself, given the circumstances!).

You have many, many cheering fans at the sidelines.

Requests to join the website pour in. Within a few days, there are over 200 community members on the Robin's Cancer Olympics site.

Many respond with gratitude for such a private social-networking service that allows them to keep up with how I am doing, to express their support, and to volunteer their help.

This Site
posted by Debbie M-M at Tuesday, June 8, 2010, 5:14 PM

> Robin: Thinking of you—knowing you are strong and you can beat this—love the web site—what a great communications tool—we all get the same message—no filters, no misinformation flying around.

One of my first Robin's Cancer Olympics (or RCO) tasks is to post under the Resources tab a pdf copy of the Perfect Storm document I had given my cancer treatment providers. Members of the RCO community, both online and in person, approach me to express their shock, sorrow, and disgust at learning of my assessment story.

Sending Cancer-fighting and Robin-loving Vibes
posted by Lesley H at Tuesday, June 15, 2010, 1:08 PM

> I am thinking of you today as you start your treatments, wishing for you to experience peace and wellbeing while the treatment helps you to fight the cancer.

> I just got on this site, so I have just read your story.

> What can I say? I am appalled and enraged at how this happened to you. I am also inspired by and applaud your courage and ability to focus on what matters most right now—you regaining health.

> I will keep you in my thoughts and prayers today and keep checking in and sending you the green, green energy of health.

Going for it!
posted by Marilyn C at Wednesday, June 9, 2010, 11:09 PM

> Wow, Robin, I just read your assessment story. I am stunned by it and a little at a loss for words (relative to my normal state...*S*). I sometimes sing at weddings. They say that if something goes wrong in the rehearsal, the wedding will go off perfectly. Sounds like you had enough errors to cover the whole first leg of your

journey. Maybe that's an omen for clear sailing from here on in. Simple math averages…

You are officially in my prayers!

The Perfect Storm
posted by Sarah C at Monday, July 12, 2010, 10:21 AM

I have just finished reading your account of the Perfect Storm and through the tears I write in praise of your courage, gutsy determination, and thoughtfulness! Those same qualities brought about the Kings Early Years Screening for School project and many other successful community initiatives. As a member of this beautiful community, I wanted to say "Thank You." Your energy, bravery, and ever-increasing optimistic take on life is contagious, dear lady.

Cheering you on to the finish line, Robin…cancer-free, hugging your family, and eating burgers once again!!

Go Robeano Go
posted by Lorraine L at Wednesday, June 9, 2010, 9:08 PM

I'm cheering for you!!!

(And I'm also feeling very disappointed in, and somewhat ashamed of, my profession after having read your Assessment History)

Robin's Cancer Olympics is launched.

6

BECOMING A CANCER PATIENT REQUIRES SUBTRACTION OF all your identities. For decades I had been "Dr. McGee"—a professional identity that I prized. So much hard work lay behind that label. But my cancer will take this away. I must now become an invalid—a patient, a number, a statistic. When my treating staff call me "Mrs." or "Ms.," I know not to correct them. Insisting on my laurels seems somehow pathetic to me. Instead, I will become "Honey"—the tag used by the nurses and technicians I encounter. I must leave my work. Maybe I will never work again.

My work as a clinical psychologist with the school board has entailed consultation to schools regarding students with behavioural or mental health issues. I meet with my school board colleagues to determine how my duties and responsibilities will be surrendered to others. I watch as my fellow psychologists resignedly take on my cases. I ache with helpless guilt. *They are already so burdened.* Some aspects of my work will simply stop, and the children and youth will do without. After 20 years, my public career as a psychologist is ended.

Over and above my public sector job, I have maintained a small private practice. My greatest concern has yet to be faced. *How do I tell my private practice patients about what has happened?*

My practice is limited to psychotherapy, mostly with adults. Although I only see three patients a week, I had been practicing that way for nearly 15 years. Consequently, I have many long-term patients, and some with very significant and serious diagnoses. Several of my patients are in the middle of complex treatment protocols for severe trauma. Eye Movement Desensitization Reprocessing Therapy, or EMDR, is a treatment that requires the patient to very slowly and carefully reprocess the traumatic memory—it is not something that could be interrupted. Sadly and ironically, I am seeing several patients for cancer-related bereavement. I am deeply concerned with the impact of my imminent departure on my private patients, particularly the very vulnerable.

During my graduate years, I had been schooled in an approach to therapy that emphasized very firm boundaries with clients. Self-disclosure was something I had almost never done. *Should I tell them? How will I handle their reactions? And mine?*

I know that in small town Nova Scotia, word gets around. *What if my private patients learn the truth before I can tell them myself?* I know that my cancer treatment will oblige me to continuously wear a slow infusion bottle clearly labeled "chemotherapy." Those patients requiring a few more sessions to finish therapy will clearly see it.

I am currently the President of my professional association, the Association of Psychologists of Nova Scotia (APNS). There are only a few weeks left in my term, after which I would normally stay on the executive as Past President. *I guess I can't do that either.*

The day I learned my diagnosis, criminals had broken into the APNS office and stolen the computer. Our Executive Director Susan Marsh is managing the aftermath of that crisis when I call her. She braces up under my news and becomes focused and helpful, as I knew she would. I ask her if she knows any other psychologist in Nova Scotia who has undergone cancer and had to close a practice.

I am in the hospital parking lot when I am called back. Susan has found someone: a senior psychologist who had experienced cancer in the past—same cancer, same stage. My mentor urges me to be forthright with all my patients. She wisely counsels me to anticipate that my patients will show a range of reactions. "They will surprise you," she says.

I make three lists: those who can be redirected by phone, those who need a personal session to prepare for transfer to a new therapist, and those I can reasonably finish with within a few weeks.

Now for the phone calls.

I am able to reach the patients on my waiting list, those with whom I had only met once, and those whose return appointments are far into the future. I tell them that I need to close my practice for "health reasons." It is difficult to hear the note of curiosity and bewilderment in their voices; however, most are satisfied with the list of alternative therapists I provide.

The personal sessions are more difficult. I enter into each of those sessions, greeting the patient as always. As the session unfolds, I feel the weight of my unsaid words. *I have to leave this person*, I think sorrowfully. *But I want them to know I would never abandon them for any lesser reason.*

When I get the words out, I am surprised by many of my patients' reactions. Instead of crumbling or crying or becoming angry, most are wonderful. Some react with genuine shows of affection ("But I love you!" one cries, as she jumps from the chair to hug me). Some are stunned and need several repetitions of my news to absorb it. Some respond with a kind of sober awe. Some patients announce with confidence that they are well enough to wait the many years it may take for me to recover. *My mentor was right*, I marvel. Many of those I thought would fall apart are strong and brave. I am genuinely touched and impressed with the degree of compassion and maturity my patients demonstrate, even though it feels so odd to be on the receiving end of their concern.

Colleagues who have heard of my plight have offered to take on the patients I must transfer. Each patient agrees to the transfer I have arranged. During a joint session with the new therapist, we say goodbye. We are both shaken. Nevertheless, their relief and mine is palpable, and our partings are dignified by the warmth and support of the incoming therapist. I am so grateful that my charges will be cared for, but so sorry to leave them nonetheless.

I have one last responsibility. I must finish the therapy protocols of a few patients who are very close to the end of their treatment.

ROBIN McGEE

Most are trauma patients. I am worried about how things will go. *Will they feel they need to take care of me and hence not be forthcoming with their issues? Will they consider their own issues to be insignificant against what they know of mine? Will I truly be able to focus on them, given my own distress and preoccupation?*

Fortunately, I have very clear treatment plans with my remaining patients. To my relief, each one is able to adopt a focused approach to their final sessions. I will be able to embark on my daily radiation treatments with a clear conscience and a clear schedule.

I cry as I walk to the parking lot for the last time. I may never practice psychology again. It has been one of the proud purposes of my life, but now it is over. I am only 48, and my life as a working person has ended.

Word of my illness has spread throughout our community like wildfire. Former patients contact me to offer me concrete help: lawn-mowing, food, drives to medical appointments. I do not know how to field their kind, well-meaning offers of tangible help. *Would accepting such help cross important boundaries better left in place? Would they be injured or hurt if I refused their assistance? Would I deprive them of a meaningful act of closure or respect?*

Maybe I can come up with alternative arms-length gestures that seem appropriate. If I can match these gestures to a meaningful aspect of the patient's therapy with me, perhaps we can both find healing. One of my patients had identified "70s music" as a resource and a "safe place" for himself during his work with me. When he offers to drive me to appointments, I ask him instead if he would make me a CD of his favourite 70s music.

"That way," I tell him, "when we each listen to it, you can think of me getting better, and I can think of you getting better."

I come home from a medical appointment to find that my lawn has been mowed by a former patient, who has left a note explaining her good deed. In my mailbox I find several homemade, crudely constructed "get well" cards from several of my child patients. Touched and grateful, I hold them against my heart.

....

We wait for treatment to start, but the tumour is not waiting. The pain is mounting: an intense aching pressure spreads throughout my abdomen.

It has been three days without any bowel movement. The tumour is bleeding more copiously now. The Nova Scotia Cancer Centre allows patients to call and leave a message to report problems. Increasingly desperate and afraid, I call to describe my situation.

When my nurse Cara returns my call, she says she has checked with Dr. Bahl. My blockage is likely mechanical, he has told her. The tumour is obstructing me. He will arrange for me to have an emergency X-ray at my local hospital.

Dr. Bahl calls back in person that afternoon.

"The X-ray shows you have seven days of digestion that has not made it through your system," he says. "Your tumour is now so large that it may block you completely. If that should happen, you will require emergency surgery—an emergency permanent colostomy. You may need that in the next 24 hours or the next few days. Your tumour is so low that it will not result in the vomiting typical with intestinal obstruction. Rather, you will experience significant pain and abdominal distension. If you do not have the surgery, you would be in danger of bowel rupture, which can be fatal. I want you to go on a liquid diet *starting now.*"

The other phone rings as Dr. Bahl is talking. It is the surgeon Dr. McIntyre's office. "You better take that," Dr. Bahl urges, "and ask about that emergency surgery."

I am shivering as I take the phone. It is Leslie Snide, Dr. McIntyre's administrative assistant, calling to reschedule an appointment. Bewildered, I describe to Leslie what I have just heard from Dr. Bahl. I am so stunned that I am wandering in my description—I do not grasp the significance of what I am saying to her.

Leslie has worked for Dr. McIntyre for 14 years. She listens sagaciously to my naive ramblings. Instantly perceiving the danger I am in, she reassures me calmly that she will slot me in to see him tomorrow. "He will know exactly what to do," she says easily.

I wait for the terrible pain. It does not come. I check my watch each hour. *Another hour of survival,* I think. Andrew paces the house anxiously. When Austin comes home from school and hears the news, he hugs me to him wordlessly, his face a rictus of fear and helplessness.

We lie awake all night. All of us, awake. I have a bag by my bedside packed for the emergency room.

As harrowing as our news is, I still hope to find some humour in it. I ask the RCO community to pray for poop.

TREATMENT DATES AND ONGOING STRUGGLES
posted by Robin McGee, Wednesday, June 9, 2010, 5:30 PM

Hello Everyone:

Today was a trying day. Good news and bad news. Good news—the chemo and radiation start date is set for 15 June. Can't wait.

The other good news—the surgeon will see me tomorrow now. This man is reputed to be the best surgeon in the province. "Technically perfect," other doctors and nurses tell me.

The bad news—my radiation oncologist is increasingly concerned about the risk of intestinal blockage. Today's X-ray showed that the tumour is close to "closing off" my bowel. The radiation can fix this within a few days, but I will have a scary weekend. If it blocks altogether in the next few days, I am looking at an emergency surgery. Everyone pray for poop!

To which members responded on the Lotsa Helping Hands site with support and humour:

Poop
posted by Valorie R at Wednesday, June 9, 2010, 9:11 PM

Hi Robin—

I also participated in the relay team of 5FU and a cocktail of other chemo drugs along with radiation—I know why they call it FU! I think I won the gold medal because I am here 16 years later—I always pray for POOP! Poop is a good thing.

Thank You
posted by Colleen R at Thursday, June 10, 2010, 8:35 AM

I just wanted to thank you for allowing all of us to be part of your support system.

I also want you to know I will be visualizing poop for the rest of the week/weekend, just for you.

Poop and healing vibes.

Poop
posted by Joelle C at Thursday, June 10, 2010, 8:39 PM

I have never prayed for poop before, but rest assured, I am doing so now!!!

Bill H < 6/13/2010 11:13 PM >

Our 8- and 10-year-old boys sure thought it was cool to be praying for someone to poop!

Sending you much love.

Rita V < 6/10/2010 9:48 AM >

Dear Robin:

I'm praying, girl, for lots of good shit!!! To happen!!

Helen W < 6/9/2010 6:19 PM >

Praying for poop has commenced in Carp, Ontario.

Mark says (and I am sorry), "We hope you take a Carp Dump"—it's a local thing—we live about five miles from it.

Seriously, we're hoping all goes well for you over the next few days. We are monitoring the site for updates. It's very cool.

X

....

We have heard many things about Dr. McIntyre. Nurses who have worked with him are emphatic about his extraordinary competence. "Being in the hands of Bernie McIntyre," says one retired OR nurse, "is the closest thing a patient can get to being in the hands of God." Another tells us that in her 22 years working in the Intensive Care Unit, she has never seen a patient of his admitted there. "He has certainly rescued patients from ICU," she said, "but his surgical patients never need us." I have been warned that he also has a reputation for being "gruff," "blunt," and "abrupt." I do not care at all about that. As I had told patients of my own for many years, what counts in a medical specialist is their expertise. "They are prescribing for you, not marrying you," I had said to those patients who feared that the psychiatrist would not be personable enough.

I am ushered into the sigmoid clinic, into his presence. I meet a clean, clear-eyed stocky man in his 50s who looks every inch the professional surgeon: white coat, healthy tan, clipped hair, straightforward manner.

"Rectal cancer," he says, consulting the referral letter in front of him. "Why did it take so long to diagnose you?"

"I saw four doctors," I reply. "They all missed it." I remember Dr. Four's dismissive last words. "They didn't consider it because I was under 50."

Dr. McIntyre grimaces. "Those doctors need to remember that anyone, at any age, can get cancer." He shakes his head. "Besides, the screening guidelines we use now state that those with an immediate family history, like you, should be scoped starting at 40."

I anxiously relate what I had been told about the recent X-ray and the warning that I might need an emergency colostomy. Within seconds, I am bent forward over his examination table, while he and his nurse prepare me for the sigmoid scope.

I am back in my chair afterwards. Dr. McIntyre shakes his head as he snaps off his gloves. He gestures angrily at the examination table.

"I don't know why none of those doctors could find that tumour," he says, his voice edged with contempt. "It is right there. I can touch it easily."

He washes his hands and turns to face me.

"You certainly have a very large tumour. Very large, almost all the way around. But I think you can avoid an emergency colostomy… you have just enough healthy tissue to manage that. I think you have an impaction—all the stool that cannot get past the tumour has pressed up behind it. But I think you are still wide enough to get all that out. You just have to turn it all to liquid."

He crosses one foot before the other and leans on the desk with one hand. "So this is what you should do: go to the store and buy many Fleet enemas. Use one every day. Try to hold it in for as long as you can—an hour if possible. Stand on your head if you have to. From now on, eat only liquids, no solid food at all. In fact, you should have been on a liquid diet from the day a tumour that dangerously close to obstruction was seen. Drink a glass of GoLyte—the preparation people use to get cleaned out before colonoscopies—every night. If you do those things, I think you can save yourself. You do not want surgery now, even if it means getting the cancer out. Your chances of survival are better if you can get the chemoradiation treatment to shrink the tumour first. When radiation starts, the tumour may swell initially, so you will need to stick with the GoLyte and liquid diet until it gives evidence of shrinking. That can take a few days, even up to three weeks."

I close my eyes. My head swims in unmitigated relief. *He knows what to do.*

I hold out my copy of The Perfect Storm. "You wondered why it took so long…this is why," I offer. "I am asking all my cancer treatment providers to read it."

He waves it away. "I don't need to read that," he says. "I know what you've got."

His nurse Lois takes it from me. She sinks into a chair as she reads it. When she looks up, her face is stricken.

"This is the worst thing I have ever heard," she says with slow astonishment. "It is like a comedy of errors, only nothing about this is funny."

Dr. McIntyre resumes. With practiced authority, he reviews what is to come. "Six weeks after your chemoradiation, I will be operating on you to remove your entire rectum, from here"—he points to a poster image of the internal organs—"to here. Your cancer is very large, but also high enough that I think I can reattach you to your sphincter. I think I can spare you a permanent colostomy, and give you instead a temporary ileostomy. That means you will excrete out from your small intestine, out of a little hole I will fashion for you. You will wear a bag over it. And then after you are done your months of chemo, I will reverse the ileostomy."

He nods towards the Perfect Storm document, still clutched in Lois's hand. "And I will take that," he adds gently, "and put it on your file."

Andrew is allowed to join us. Dr. McIntrye repeats his advice to my shaken husband. While he speaks, a new sad thought forms in my mind. *Dr. Four had seen an obvious obstructing tumour during my scope, and she did not tell me about it for another eight days.* I have eaten normally since my scope because I did not know not to. *Maybe this crisis could have been avoided.*

As we trudge down the hall as we leave, Lois runs after us.

"I want you to know something," she says earnestly. "Dr. McIntyre is the best. The very best. And if you end up with emergency surgery, please call him. He cares so much for his patients that even if he did not do the surgery himself, he would still like to visit you."

She reaches out to touch my shoulder. "You are finally in good hands," she breathes. "Finally."

7

I FOLLOW DR. MCINTYRE'S ADVICE TO THE LETTER. EACH day, I prop myself upside down against the bathroom wall, trying to balance on my shoulders for my hour-long enemas. I learn quickly and miserably that enemas are best done in a bathtub.

Every colorectal cancer patient eventually has to deal with excrement. Lots of it. A natural function that had never been a problem to me before is now an inexorable daily focus. As I stare up at my feet, I think about all the words we use for bowel movements: poo, poop, poopie, droppings, shit, shite, scat, kaka, logs, dump, dung, stool, feces, bung, number two, diaper dumplings, and twin boys at the pool.

I post:

STILL LIVING

posted by Robin McGee, Friday, June 11, 2010, 4:15 PM

Hello Everyone:

I seem to be still alive. What a relief!

It was a beautiful June day today—lovely in the way only the Annapolis Valley can be. We went for a ride in the 65 Herald convertible to buy more poop products. We stopped for an ice cream. Tonight there are fireworks in my town, and we may go to those. It was nice to have a day without utterly harrowing news.

Tonight Austin is helping out at the Canadian Cancer Society event "Relay for Life." I think it will do him a world of good to see many cancer survivors. He and two friends are sleeping out overnight in a tent. They call themselves "The Three Cancer-Fighting Amigos." I am so glad for his supportive friends.

I AM SO HUNGRY!!! This liquid diet is for the birds. Do they make liquid burgers?

BIG DAY TOMORROW...AND EGGS!!
posted by Robin McGee, Monday, June 14, 2010, 1:45 PM

Hi All:

Tomorrow is the big day when I finally get my chemo and radiation started. Yahoo!!

And in other good news, today they said I could add scrambled eggs to my mushy rice noodles. It is not a burger (drool), but it is a start. Those who know my ravenous appetite will appreciate what a joy this is to me.

For all community members on the Paddy's Ravens Soccer Team, please know that tomorrow I plan to wear the MVP T-shirt you gave me after the provincials a few years ago. I have treasured it so much I have never worn it! I want to wear it as a symbol of the "digging deep" one must do when playing three games of soccer in a row...Pass this on to our other teammates.

Tomorrow I will post a picture of me with my new chemo bottle. I am a brunette now. My hairdresser advised going back to my natural colour. I will retain my hair, but as you are not allowed to colour hair during chemo, we wanted it to grow out looking natural. I feel a little smarter already!

For the past 14 years, I have played Ladies 7-Aside Soccer. When my soccer teammates hear about me wearing my Most Valuable Player shirt to my first treatment, they respond warmly.

It is conventional at the end of our games to cheer the other team ("Three Cheers for the Wizards! Hip Hip Hooray!").

"And One for Robin!"
posted by Janice P at Thursday, June 10, 2010, 10:30 PM

Hey Robin,

Glad to have a chance to connect with you over this site. Thanks for setting us all up to help support you!

I am wondering if you have been feeling extra powerful surges of support, love, and encouragement on Sundays and Wednesdays, say around 6 or 7ish?...Our Ravens are now ending our end-of-game cheer with "and one for Robin!" Pat's idea, I believe, and I just love it. We are all missing you on the field but are ready in any way to help you win these Olympics.

You
posted by Monique C at Sunday, July 19, 2010, 2:15 PM

Robin...I read your messages today and I have to say I am in awe of your strength. I have seen it on the soccer field where nobody is going to get in your way...This will not either, I can see that. Every game, we say a cheer for you. Heather Miles leads it and it is a natural part of every outing now. We are thinking about you and will continue to cheer you on.

MVP Always!
posted by Monica C at Monday, June 14, 2010, 5:34 PM

Robin...glad to finally join this great site and keep up with how you are doing. I miss you terribly on the field and sure wish you were there beside me, but we are all beside you now in thought and prayer. Best of luck tomorrow—can't go wrong with your MVP shirt on!

Wear it Well

posted by Janice P at Monday, June 14, 2010, 3:38 PM

> I will be thinking of you as you start your treatments tomorrow. I
> can't believe you've never worn that shirt…Looks like you were
> saving it for the right time and tomorrow sounds perfect. Be strong
> like you are on the field!

As I read their responses, I reflect on the many analogies there
are between playing soccer and fighting cancer. All the endurance it requires, the challenge of determining the greatest threat,
and needing to turn on a dime as conditions change. As a defence
player, I had learned that sometimes the ball-carrier will surrender
the ball if you challenge her. To become an obstacle to her and to
hang on like a bulldog. There is no running away from cancer. No
substitutions to rest you. There is only one direction to run: directly
at it, toward it. I must *tackle* cancer.

....

I have survived the immediate threat of blockage. The chemoradiation event of my cancer Olympics is about to begin.

We pull up outside the Halifax Infirmary. This is where they are
going to put in the PICC line that will deliver my chemotherapy.

Andrew is desperately squeamish. In Grade 10, he had to be
dragged out of Science class by his heels when he fainted during
a lab in which they had to prick their fingers to get drops of blood.
He cannot enter the Halifax Infirmary with me, so sickened is he by
the prospect of a PICC line in my beating heart.

I enter an enormous operating theatre, staffed by two nurses
in OR scrubs. I lie on the table while one nurse prepares my arm.
A TV-screen looms above me. The nurses keep me talking, asking
questions about my work as a psychologist. I turn my head to the
side when they insert the lengthy catheter into my arm. An image
of my heart appears on the screen, with the bones of my ribcage in
the foreground.

Above her operating mask, the nurse's eyes swerve over to the screen. "There it is," she says. "It is in your heart now. See?"

I can make out the dark line against the grey palpitating mass.

"You have 20 minutes to make it over to the Victoria building in the other hospital. They will attach your chemo bottle there. Good luck."

Andrew shivers as I get in the car, seeing the meshing that covers the line. "You are so brave," he says, his voice catching.

We head up the elevators to the 11th floor of the Victoria Building, where the chemotherapy unit is waiting. An affable nurse escorts us to a room with four reclining chairs. She gestures for me to sit in one and pulls up closer in her castered chair.

She produces a bottle with a full plastic bladder inside it. It is about the size of a baby bottle, the word "CHEMOTHERAPY" affixed to it in red capital letters. She efficiently secures the bottle to the PICC line, swathing my tubes in tape and mesh.

"There are four things you should be careful of and that you must check for every day, " she advises. "The first is a kink in the line from the bottle to your arm. The second thing is to check that the line is open and not closed by the key clamp. The third issue is usage—the size of the balloon should visibly decrease every day. And make sure that the connector is taped to your skin. Four things I want you to review and check every day. Can you think of a way to remember those four things?"

"I need an acronym," I say, "one that uses those four elements—kinks, usage, closure, and skin..."

Andrew is punchdrunk with stress. "I know!" he exclaims. "How about SUCK!"

We dissolve in laughter, while the nurse looks on bemused.

The nurse warns us firmly about many risks: of ripping the catheter out accidently, of burning through it while cooking, of breaking the chemo bottle. She gives us several harrowing anecdotes of these things happening to patients she has known. I must not go out in sunlight: she tells a story of a man whose face swelled into blisters by merely driving for 10 minutes in a convertible. We do not impress her with our seriousness, as we keep giggling help-lessly, too horrified to absorb her lessons.

I leave with my new friend in my new woollen sling and with a "toxic spill kit" to use if the bottle ever breaks.

Now for radiation.

The radiation waiting room is crowded. I look around at my fellow cancer patients. I see the breast cancer patients, hairless and wrapped in their johnny shirts. I see the esophageal patients, with burn marks along the side of their faces and necks. Some have tra-cheotomies. I see a patient who has no nose behind the mask she wears. Several patients are being brought in on gurneys by ambu-lance attendants. I overhear the poignant conversations among the weathered working class men from the farms, dockyards, and mines of Nova Scotia.

"They never gave us no protection," one says to another, "not a mask or anything, working with that stuff all day."

I drink my obligatory two glasses of water one half-hour before my appointment. When my name is called, I follow the technician into the radiation room.

The radiation machine is enormous, with large, insect-like eyes that I imagine target those powerful and invisible beams. I am told to lie face down on the table, my face held in place by a padded ring. I feel the platform raise itself and launch me slowly forward until I am under its hidden but intimidating stare.

The technicians consult a big black binder.

"That's bad, that is very bad," one of them tells the other, looking back and forth between me and the binder in her partner's hands. "When are you seeing your doctor again?" she asks me anxiously.

What is bad? Is that binder about me?

As I close my eyes, the techs surround me, tugging me into place. Previously, they have tattooed small black marks on the skin on my back and hips. These permanent pinpoints help determine the precise alignment of the radiation beams; they support consistency across multiple treatments. When the technicians are satisfied that I am finally in the right position, they step back.

"There will be three beams that will come at you from three sides, one side at a time," the head technician explains. They dash into their protective booth at the back of the room.

There is a warning sound, like a squeal, and a powerful thrum as the beam to my right begins. I feel nothing. After what feels like a few minutes, it switches off. Another thrumming begins, this time from above my back. The thrum from my left follows last. Suddenly all the equipment is silent except for the scrape and squeal of the bed lowering itself.

"That's it?" I ask as I get off the bed. "That seemed to take about 10 minutes."

"That was your first one of twenty-eight," the tech replies. 'See you tomorrow."

....

I post to the RCO blog several pictures of myself holding my chemotherapy bottle. I mug for the camera, flexing my encumbered arm like a fighter.

AND SHE'S OFF!
posted by Robin McGee, Tuesday, June 15, 2010, 6:30 PM

Hello RCO:

Today the battle was well and truly joined!

I went to get the PICC line in first. The nurses distracted me from the BIG NEEDLE by telling me about their children's psychological problems...it worked like a charm!

Then it was off to chemo to get my new friend, my 5FU bottle. It will infuse me at a tiny rate 24 hours a day. I have to sleep and bathe with it (somehow). There are pictures of me with it on the Photo Gallery tab.

Does anyone on this list get the Chronicle Herald newspaper delivered? They recommended that I collect the long plastic bags the paper is delivered in to use as shower-protection for the chemo bottle and tubes. Save your bags!

Then it was off to Radiation. I had to lay down on my front with my head in a "rest oval"—just like at a massage therapist. Because I am facing down, I cannot see what is happening, only hear it. It sounds awesome—whirring, powerful, profound. Just what you would think the power of the sun would sound like.

I am so glad that the cavalry has now arrived to help my immune cells fight this thing! I think of these treatments like one thinks of the Allies invading on D-Day—as liberators. When others fret about my normal cells, I think that compares to someone complaining that the Allied tanks ripped up their lawn on the way to fighting the Nazis.

Tomorrow is more radiation and chemo check-in, and Thursday is radiation plus doctor. More later!

Patricia B < 6/15/2010 7:50 PM >

Rawbean,

Are you supposed to carry that chemo bottle cosy thing around under your clothes? In your purse or backpack? Or is it jewelry?

Is that your MVP shirt you're wearing in the pictures? If so, I think the lettering should be much bigger...

Have you seen the movie *The Devil Wears Prada*? There's a part about "girding one's loins" for the onslaught ahead (e.g., arrival of evil boss) that reminds me of what you did today. I am awed by you. And teaching others how to distract you is brilliant—I can try that during my upcoming oral surgery (although not being able to ask questions is a drawback).

It's so good to get frequent updates on your situation—it helps us all go day by day and live in the moment. If I know you're okay today, I don't have to worry about you until tomorrow.

The doorbell rings repeatedly. Several community members have already responded to my post. They come bearing dozens of pink plastic Chronicle Herald sleeves.

When it is time to shower, I sit on the bed while Andrew tugs the pink plastic over my apparatus. He has found a Velcro knee brace that clasps the bottle firmly against my forearm. I watch his face solemnly. His brows are knit with concentration as he finds a way to protect all the bottles, mesh, and tubes underneath the plastic.

I used to be an independent contributor to the household. I used to do so much—all the groceries, childcare, yard work. Now, I am dependent on Andrew for my most basic personal care.

The words of the Anglican marriage service come to my mind, the vows we had taken 20 years before.

...to have and to hold from this day forward,

Andrew will have to leave his job. He was at the top of his career arc—a senior manager in an engineering consulting firm. He was responsible for millions of dollars in projects and dozens of staff. Now, he will cease his work life as suddenly as I left mine. He will take an indefinite leave to stay home to look after me.

For better, for worse,

His life will become a nightmare, as will mine. Once again, he will be plunged into anguish, so soon after caring for his terminally ill father over the past year.

For richer, for poorer,

When my sick leave runs out, I will be forced to go on Long Term Disability. Andrew must take sick time and leave without pay. Even with public health care, we know that this cancer will cost us many hundreds of thousands.

In sickness and in health,

Andrew will cook all our meals, now that I must not. He will drive me to all my appointments, because I can no longer drive myself.

To love and to cherish for the rest of our lives,
according to God's holy law.

He carefully secures the tape to my skin.

This is my solemn vow.

Andrew pats my shoulder as he completes his nursing task. His blue eyes twinkle as he looks up at me. He playfully hums the theme to "Polythene Pam" from the Beatles' *Abbey Road* album.

We both burst out laughing.

The chemoradiation event has begun.

8

As the weeks of radiation unfold, I find myself confronting the challenges that each cancer patient must face. Other people, other medical ideas.

I need to adjust from being a private citizen to a public tragic figure. When people in the street hail me with "How are you?" I have to search their faces. *Do they know? Have they heard?* There is always a moment of awkwardness when encountering someone I have not seen recently—which Robin would he or she respond to?

Some people know that cancer is like a car accident: it can happen to anyone. Most people respond to me with equanimity and concern, and sometimes with respectful awe. But the sheer anxiety of the word "cancer" propels others into awkward and sometimes unusual pronouncements. Some crow about their own health or the thoroughness of their doctors with a kind of frightened defence. Many abjure me that I must, at all costs, remain "positive." If I allow myself to feel negative emotions, these would thwart treatment and hasten my death. I wondered how many people would give such advice to soldiers heading to war.

So many well-meaning people, in a fumbling effort to relate, say things that are puzzling at best and terrifying at worst. "Oh, colorectal cancer...my uncle had that. He was diagnosed on Monday and dead by Friday." "I heard your news, and it made me feel wonderful that I am not you." "Would you like to see this obituary? It was from a brave woman much younger than you with the same diagnosis." "My friend had the same cancer as you, and at first he responded to treatment but it came back and he died in agony... *agony!*" Some want me to read the poetry and prose of the valiant cancer dead, including their piteous prayers for a never-seen recovery. Some want me to read and watch *The Last Lecture*, in which a professor with pancreatic cancer demonstrates that he can do one-arm push ups—only to die two months later. Literature that helps the healthy to remember their mortality and stand in awe of life is not helpful to me. I am plenty aware of my mortality.

I try to be patient with all these responses. I remember from my infertility days that many people say stupid things to the afflicted ("Just relax and you will have a baby"). I understand these words as clumsy attempts to connect. In any case, the sheer weight of cancer prevents me from taking these remarks too seriously. No words, whether kindly or cruelly meant, could ever change the fact that I am deep, deep in the mud pit.

I am bombarded with advice about alternative medicine: macrobiotic diet, antioxidants, naturopathy, juicing, Reiki, reflexology—the list is endless and overwhelming. I cannot choose between any of them. The oncology team has warned me against antioxidants during chemo. They tell me that cancer cells can "hide" behind antioxidants, which will protect them just as much as their normal cell counterparts. So I hold off on all such interventions, putting my faith in conventional medicine. I have so much to learn, even with regard to ordinary treatments.

I seek books that can help me and calm me. *Love, Medicine and Miracles* was written by surgeon Dr. Bernie Siegel in 1986. It is commonly regarded as the seminal work that inspired modern understanding of the mind-body connection in oncology. Dr. Siegel posited that cancer patients had better outcomes if they had certain characteristics: the will to live, the verve to search for the best care, and a benign perspective on their treatments. Often, he said, cancer patients are told that radiation and chemotherapy are destructive and poisonous. Patients become brainwashed by such messages, and suffer undue anxiety. Rather, he suggested, patients ought to see radiation as the harnessed power of the sun and the universe in a coherent ray, beaming down upon them to heal the cancer. Chemotherapy is not poison to a cancer patient—it is the elixir of life. Dr. Siegel advocated meditation, visualization, exercise, and spiritual approaches as adjuncts to medical therapies. This book offers me some solace: it underscores the truth that some cancer patients do live, and that perhaps I could be one of them. Many of the characteristics of positive-outcome patients I already had, such as will and verve. As a psychologist, I was already familiar with the positive impacts of exercise, meditation, and visualization on well-being.

So each day, as I climb upon the radiation table, I visualize the power of the stars as the instrument thrums to life. When the pitched hum of the machine tells me that the beams are entering me, I imagine the tumour cringing and melting like the Wicked Witch of the West. I imagine that my inner passages are opening up. Somehow, that sensation lasts even after the treatment is over.

The liquid diet is punishing. I am ravenous and weak, and I fear my weakness. I have six weeks of chemotherapy and radiation before me, and I dread facing those challenges debilitated by hunger. I will be permitted something more than fluids and mush only as the radiation decreases the size and imminent lethality of my tumour. The RCO community is supportive, at once humourous and sympathetic.

TODAY'S IMPROVEMENTS
posted by Robin McGee, Wednesday, June 16, 2010, 6:15 PM

Hello All:

Today I feel oddly better. Maybe the treatments are working already, or maybe it is because I ate HALF A TUNA SANDWICH!! I just had a reasonable mashed supper too. Please Sir, can I have some more?

Today I had my PICC line adjusted and another dose of radiation. Last night I learned to sleep with my new bottle attachment—no problem so far. Showering is another matter. I look like Frankenrobin, with taped-up plastic sheathes covering my tubes and bottle. Now that is a picture I WILL NOT put on the RCO website Photo Gallery!

Anyone for a broth smoothie?

Sharon R < 6/18/2010 8:33 PM >

If you say I could have a broth and cheerios smoothie with you, Robin, let's set a date!!!

Judy K < 6/14/2010 2:23 PM >

Oh Robin!

God love you—you are so funny !!!!!!!

Good luck with chemo and radiation—you will be a trooper.

Enjoy your eggs—maybe they'll come up with hamburger-flavored rice noodles.

Be good at that hospital tomorrow—kick ASS big time.

Liquid Diet Doldrums
posted by Beth R on Friday, June 11, 2010

Remember also, Robin, that your Olympic events do not include the 100-metre sprint as you grab a burger off someone's barbeque and scarf it down in that record-breaking 100-m dash!

While awaiting the return of more substance foodwise, you can create your own dream menu! Seems to be an oral fixation. :)

Liquids
posted by Tara S at Saturday, June 12, 2010, 8:36 AM

Liquids aren't all bad...and an oral fixation is perhaps better than the alternative fixations...

Marla D < 6/16/2010 8:55 PM >

Yummm tuna!!! When can you do steak?

Glad you and the bottle are getting along so well. When will they put something more interesting in it? (I was thinking Kahlua would be nice!)

I am thinking of you—will it soon be time for tea or a walk???

Keep the emails coming (I am enjoying the photos too, but thanks for not sharing the one in the shower!!)

Several others send stories of their own experiences with a liquid diet...what it was like to fall ravenously upon a plate of mashed potatoes with butter after having a jaw wired shut, what it was like to bite down on a soft-boiled egg after weeks of broth and jello.

The radiation techs have encouraged me to use aloe vera on my skin, directly from the plant. They tell me to ensure air circulation around the burnt bum—on their advice, I start wearing skirts without underwear. I attach a small fan to the foot of my bed, so air can be directed at my reddening skin. The fan is required for another reason—to quell the emergence of the disabling hot flashes, the signal of my new, sudden, profound, and artificial menopause, resulting from the slow destruction of my ovaries.

SATURDAY AT LAST
posted by Robin McGee, Saturday, June 19, 2010, 9:00 AM

Hello Readers:

Today I am enjoying my first cup of coffee in a week. Bliss out!

Yesterday I went in to my appointment with my friend and colleague Daphne, who is herself a cancer survivor. She was going for her regular checkup. Her appointment was morning and mine was not till late afternoon, so I was able to fit in two meetings: one with a dietician and the other with the Association of Psychologists of Nova Scotia! I am now Past President of APNS, having been President right up until last month.

The dietician was interesting. She affirmed that I will want to stay on a minimum residue diet and gave me ideas for that. She also explained that cancer patients need far more calories than most people. "Whatever you did about calories before," she said, "do the opposite now." This means slathering potatoes in butter and sour cream, putting whipped cream on everything, and consuming as much pudding and cheesecake as one can scarf. Meat protein will still be minimal for me for awhile—I can have one soft-cooked piece of chicken a week (*sob*). However, I can have peanut butter, hummus, and soft cheese. Surprisingly, despite all my hardships, I have not lost any weight. She was delighted by this, as she says it means I was able to meet my caloric needs with the Ensure. Perhaps most important—I CAN HAVE COFFEE AGAIN! SLURP!

APNS was good as well. It was great to see my colleagues there again, and to spend even a little time doing something normal. It was very productive and satisfying.

Afterwards I went back to the hospital for the radiation. I am not sure how many people feel this way, but I LOVE radiation. For me, it feels like going to the massage therapist. As soon as I get off the table, I feel better. It feels as if the tumour is melting away afterwards, which it is.

I may not always feel this good, but right now, I actually feel better than I did a week ago. Maybe it is the psychological relief of starting treatment, or maybe it is the body's joyful response to the destruction of a potentially lethal enemy. My tumour would have killed me mechanically, even if it never metastasized, so feeling it diminish is so very welcome. So far, no side effects of either chemo or radiation.

Hope everyone is enjoying the day, wherever you are.

Sharon R < 6/19/2010 4:29 PM >

There are some things to be said about coffee, Robin. Hit the cheesecake hard!!!

Thea B < 6/21/2010 8:18 AM >

Man! You're not being a very good cancer patient. You're supposed to be telling us harrowing tales of how awful it is to be sick, so we will all feel better about our lives and heap mounds of pity on you!

I'M SO GLAD! You are an inspiration.

I cannot be around food. At dinnertime, when Andrew and Austin are having their meals, I must escape. I walk the countryside with my friend Pam and her aged dog Julie. Pam's boisterous manner conceals a deep sensitivity, and her companionship is a balm.

As we walk, I swing a left arm encumbered by my bottle and its wrappings. The woollen bottle holder has proven too painful to wear, as the fibres scrape my neck raw. Andrew, ever the innovator, adapts an old fanny pack that allows me to wear the bottle at my waist.

Walking serves as a reminder that I can still take steps—literally steps—towards wellness. I reflect that my body is still my ally. It has not betrayed me; rather, it has been besieged by an enemy while the guards were sleeping. I try with my mind to send my body a message: *you and I are in this together, as friends.*

....

Each day, the members of the RCO community send astonishing and warm messages, channelling to me a love and respect I did not know I had earned.

HAPPY FATHER'S DAY

posted by Robin McGee, Sunday, June 20, 2010, 4:30 PM

Happy Father's Day to All:

Another positive day with no side effects. I can feel that my tumour has shrunk already...I feel more "open."

Today I had a very positive time at my private practice, which I will be wrapping up before July. I feel very grateful for all my psychology colleagues, who have offered to take on my patients, and to the patients themselves, who have been remarkable in their warmth and understanding.

Yesterday Andrew prepared a special e-book with photos for his own father. It was very, very touching. Ron is dying at his home in the islands, as was his wish. Andrew wants to convey to Ron the impact Ron has had on his life. Please pray that Ron will be well enough to read it, and that it gives him pleasure and peace.

I hope all of you are enjoying or remembering your own fathers today, or are out being good fathers yourselves.

Roger and Joan B < 6/20/2010 8:09 PM >

This morning, you and I ran the Johnny Miles Half Marathon together in New Glasgow. I ran it literally, you figuratively. I was reminded of the women in India who work treadmills to generate electricity and carbon credits for others who need them. So I determined to generate energy and endorphins for YOU towards your Cancer Olympics.

In a moment of selfishness, I wondered if I sent all the endorphins your way, would I crash and fail to complete the 21 kilometres? But then the Holy Spirit reminded me that despite your brilliant success in maintaining your weight, "you ain't heavy—you're my sister." So, on I ran.

At about 16k, I thought I might "hit the wall," but I could hear your voice screaming "faster, faster!" right beside me. At that point, I recalled how competitive you are in soccer, so I determined not to wimp out and walk. We finished running! Lots of energy and lots of endorphins directed to your Olympic effort.

Robin, I was so touched to hear about Andrew's e-book for Ron. They are both in my prayers.

Have a wonderful week, sister!

ANOTHER DAY, ANOTHER ZAP
posted by Robin McGee, Monday, June 21, 2010, 4:30 PM

Hello All:

Today was our first straightforward day—drive in, radiation, drive out. This week's appointments are nearly all at noon, which allows for not much else in the day. This getting well is a full-time job!

Speaking of jobs, I am sending out my bliss vibes to all you teachers out there. Only a few more days to go and you will all be free. Put on Louis Armstrong's "Summertime," break out the beer and the hammock, and RELAX!!

Andrew's father Ron was able to read his e-book: thank you for all those prayers. He is asleep much of the time now, hopefully in comfort.

Today I received a message from my dear friend Joan who ran a half-marathon in my honour yesterday. I am very, very touched and honoured by these gestures of respect and support—they are very healing for me.

Lesley H < 6/21/2010 5:29 PM >

Robin—

It is so great to hear how "open" you are! It is truly and deeply inspiring—when I read your emails today, I felt my own closed-off bits cracking open; it reconnected me with my own gratitude for my life and for people in my life. Thanks so much for that gift!

I am cheering you on!

We try to be stoic. We try to manage. Andrew has spent weeks turning down offers of lawn-mowing from neighbours, afraid that we would burn them out with our needs. I have a different view. I know that people want to help in concrete ways, even need to. I tell Andrew that asking for help is providing others a path to their own salvation, their own gesture aimed at redeeming and reversing the cloud of menace that surrounds us.

I post:

UNDERESTIMATION
posted by Robin McGee, Wednesday, June 23, 2010, 6:30 PM

Hello Everyone:

Today we came to the realization that we need more help than we thought. Driving in daily for radiation takes so much time that we have NO time leftover to look after the house, the chores, the lawn, etc. Trying to fit in health-related behaviors (such as resting, walking, visualization exercises, reading about recovery) has been challenging. So we have agreed that I can add more driving help to the calendar, so that Andrew can deal with cooking and recycling and Austin care at least one more day a week.

The psychology faculty at Acadia University gave me a lovely gift today! My friend Lisa Price came over to plant a Rose of Sharon, a beautiful shrub. It will grow to its ultimate size and gorgeousness in eight years...another reason to live! God bless you, Psychology Department!

I have set up the Lotsa Helping Hands website to show the chores for which we need help. I watch in astonishment. Within one hour of posting this announcement, eight people have signed up on the website calendar offering to drive me to radiation appointments. The drive is a long one—close to an hour and a half. Nevertheless, volunteers come forth from all over the region.

On those drives, we share. My drivers talk about their own hurts, losses, and health problems. They talk about dark times in their own lives, and how they overcame them. I feel the roots tying me to my community becoming deeper, drawing me further into the soil of our common heartaches, our common vistas.

As the radiation progresses, my skin becomes increasingly sensitive. RCO members come by the house with clothes—skirts for me to wear, as now I cannot wear pants or even underwear. They give me DVDs of movies and TV shows. They come by to garden. They send me CDs and MP3s of music they have found uplifting and inspirational. Some even compose music for me.

RESTFUL SATURDAY
posted by Robin McGee, Saturday, June 26, 2010, 3:45 PM

Hello All:

It is so wonderful to be able to relax on a Saturday—no treatments to rush off to. I sit and rest and dream of things to eat (hmmm... mushroom risotto is my new craving...). The BOSE system is helping me to enjoy the music some of you have sent.

I am reading the book *Anticancer: A New Way of Life*. It was written by doctor/neuroscientist David Servan-Schreiber, who discovered he had brain cancer by playing around with his own MRI research equipment. He extols the virtues of diet, emotional peace, and exercise as complements to conventional treatment. I felt anxious reading the part about diet, and had trouble sleeping afterwards. The only food I can eat now (white flour, dairy) are considered cancer-feeding culprits. But my mother-in-law wisely commented, "That is like worrying about hangnails when your hair is on fire." I have made my peace that I have to eat this minimal residue diet to keep me safe until the tumour has shrunk to a safer size.

One of the things this book says is the following: "Recent studies show, in fact, that it is not only the love of a husband, a wife, or children that can enable morale to remain strong and slow the progression of illness, but also the simple love and caring attention of friends old and new." How true this is, and how grateful I am to all of you on this website for your support.

HAPPY CANADA DAY
posted by Robin McGee, Thursday, July 1, 2010, 1:45 PM

It is a lovely Canada Day out there today. I am enjoying it from my vampirish indoor-in-the-shade perspective. It is nice to keep the windows open to at least enjoy the sounds and scents. I am also grateful for the break—treatments are not held on holidays, so I did not have to go into Halifax today.

I am trying to work towards a routine of one meal a day with some solid food. All other meals are liquid. So I am doing lots of smoothies and soups. I spend my days fantasizing about that one chewable thing—today, that will be perogies with dollops of rich yogurt...(more drool).

For entertainment, two friends gave us the first 13 episodes of the show *Glee*. We have been laughing ourselves silly watching it. It is one of those shows, like *Buffy the Vampire Slayer* or *30 Rock*, that is so funny you have to rewind it to catch all the jokes. Funny movies and series are definitely the way to go when you are sick. I am sure there is alot of research literature on that (she said, pondering psychologically).

Special thanks to all of you who have volunteered to come over on Saturday afternoon to help me with my garden. Please bring your tools for planting and weeding, as I have lots of the latter to do! Also, bring a container to take away any flowers you want—I have

lots that need dividing. I will have the snacks and ice tea ready.
Looking forward to it!

Enjoy your day!

HOT!
posted by Robin McGee, Saturday, July 10, 2010, 1:45 PM

Hello All:

Today is another hot and humid day here. We rarely put on the
AC because of concerns for the cost and environment, but today
I insisted. Today my former soccer team is playing several games
in a row in a big tournament. My heart and my waterbottle go out
to them. Memories of how much courage and effort are required to
go on in soccer under such conditions are often what I call upon
when I am rallying for my treatments.

People have asked me what the overall effects of radiation are like.
For me, it feels the way it would if you had spent a day in the hot
sun. Afterwards you are somewhat tired, warm, and thirsty. You
don't want alcohol, just water.

On Thursday, I was able to eat a piece of pizza. It was much like
that scene in the book *Eat Pray Love*, in which the main character
buys the best pizza in the world in Naples. Tears of joy course
down her face as she surrenders to the euphoria of eating it. I am
sure the people in the hospital cafeteria were astonished to see
my raptures.

Hoping you all stay cool. Tomorrow, all of us will be riveted for the
World Cup final. I have a bottle of single malt scotch wagered on
the Dutch.

RON

posted by Robin McGee, Monday, July 12, 2010, 5:30 PM

Hello All:

I make a sad announcement today: my father-in-law Ron Hurst died today, in his sleep. His wife heard his laboured breathing, around 5:30 am, and she went into his room to investigate. He was asleep. He took one more big breath, and then he was gone.

Although we are deeply saddened, I am comforted by the fact that he died as he wanted: in the islands, outside a hospital, without pain, and with his wife present. He will be cremated and his ashes spread at sea.

Andrew is understandably broken up about it. He and his siblings are thinking of how they might commemorate Ron's life in an informal but collective way, given that they are so many miles apart. As per Ron's wishes, we visited him last month—he did not want us going to the islands for a funeral. Nevertheless, I think we would all benefit from some kind of ritual way to show our respect and say goodbye. Maybe some of you have ideas from your own bereavement experiences.

The RCO community share their bereavement rituals. Many went to the sea and had private rituals on the beach. Some planted trees. Some mounted fireworks. Some had parties and sing-alongs. After much deliberation, Andrew chooses to build a model ship that he can set to sea. This idea seems to work on two levels of tribute. The sea was Ron's true home. Ron was a skilled craftsman, and model ships were a speciality of his. It also offers Andrew a means of channelling his emotions through his hands—his voice is not up to the task.

I write Ron's obituary, my face wet with tears.

I post:

TOO DARN HOT

posted by Robin McGee, Sunday, July 18, 2010, 12:00 PM

Hello Sweltering Everyone:

I hope you are all in a cool place today. It is 30 degrees in the shade here and humid too. Despite all that, I am feeling a little better. The vomiting has not recurred (maybe unrelated?) and the diarrhea is at bay today. I am pondering going to see the movie *Inception* today...maybe I will sit in the last row in the back near the aisle, just in case!

Several of you have asked me about my fear of death. Oddly, it is not death I fear. I fear suffering, and I fear bereaving my family. Death I imagine approaching as I approach everything—with curiosity and reflection. (I was a "Green" under True Colours—the curious type). Faith helps, of course. The funny thing about facing one's own death is that it seems so inconvenient! I think: I can't die now...I haven't finished reading the collected works of George Elliot! I can't die now...I haven't written the Great Canadian Novel! I can't die now...I haven't finished the final season of *Buffy the Vampire Slayer*! To all of you out there with unfinished projects, I say "Get on with it!"

Andrew is spending the weekend carefully crafting the sailing boat model for his Dad's memorial. He has to modify it so that it will be ocean-going and not just a desktop model. It is amazingly detailed. I will take a picture of it for the RCO website's Photo Gallery when it is done.

Stay Cool.

....

I do not blame God for my condition. However, neither can I bring myself to pray for my own life. It seems selfish somehow, presumptuous and unreasonable. Why should I live when people are dying in the Pakistan earthquakes in their thousands? Likewise, sudden churchgoing seems inherently wrong. If I had not been a regular attendee before, going now seems like hollow begging. God would see through that, as I do. Wise believers tell me that I am not fooling anyone by such a perspective: God already knows I want my life to be spared.

I can and do pray for strength and comfort. I need to find a way to reconnect with my spiritual self to be able to go on, to fight the gut-crushing and all-pervading dread that assails me.

I decide to search for the tenderness of worship where I had found it before: in music. I had always been drawn to the music of Bruce Cockburn. But I am also moved by classical pieces that bespeak God's grace and majesty: Bach, Handel, Beethoven, Mozart. The RCO community sends me CDs of music they find uplifting and inspirational. I put all the Bruce Cockburn songs on my ipod in shuffle mode.

One of Cockburn's songs from his early repertoire touches me as I lie down each day on the radiation table:

Lord of the Starfields
Ancient of Days
Universe Maker
Here's a song in your praise

Wings of the storm cloud
Beginning and End
You make my heart leap
Like a banner in the wind

Oh Love that fires the sun,
Keep me burning

9

EACH WEEK, I SEE DR. BAHL. HIS PRESENCE IS SOOTHING, and his bedside manner is unflappable. He patiently explains each phenomenon, listens attentively, and examines gently. Eventually, I was able to read the case summary he wrote about me. His three-page report was thoroughly and conscientiously written, so much so that later clinicians remarked on its comprehensiveness in their own reviews. Not for the first time, I marvel at how greatly physicians can differ. It seems oddly surreal to be in his considerate and considered care, after my experiences with Doctors One through Four. I often reflect that his professional and gracious manner with me is as therapeutic as any of the active treatments I am undergoing.

Astonishingly, I continue to meet with secretarial ineptitude from Dr. Three's office.

I post:

ANGRY AGAIN
posted by Robin McGee, Thursday, June 17, 2010, 9:30 PM

Hello Everyone:

Today I experienced an event that roused my anger over this whole thing again. Yesterday I called my family doctor's office to ask for copies of all my bloodwork and test results dating back to 2007. I explained that I wanted to know my health parameters from before the probable onset of the cancer, so I can know my baseline health indices. I signed the necessary releases.

I picked it up today. When I was perusing the documents a few hours later, I noticed that some of the records were missing. I called. The secretary explained that she had decided not to give me them all, just "the few that had any positive findings."

Readers, I blew a gasket. "When I say ALL my bloodwork," I yelled into the phone, "I mean ALL my bloodwork!!!" After what I have been through, it enraged me to think I still cannot trust that office.

Various members of the RCO community respond with outrage, but also with encouragement.

Angry Again!
posted by Joelle C at Thursday, June 17, 2010, 11:22 PM

Don't blame you at all for being angry, Robin. Anger can be empowering...get those records.

Every day brings more progress in the fight! We are with you.

Lesley H < 6/18/2010 8:51 AM >

It is near impossible not to get angry under these circumstances! I am angry on your behalf!

Cindy H < 6/17/2010 11:12 PM >

I cannot believe this insane story. Oh my! Since when does the secretary choose what to send and what not to send? You have EVERY RIGHT to those bloodwork reports...they are YOURS. Good for you for blowing a gasket...I blew one when I read this.

And there is honestly nothing I would rather do than share a broth smoothie with you. I adore your stamina...you daily teach me life lessons. Robin, you are amazing. You WILL beat this... keep fighting. I've got my fists in the air every time I think about the things you deal with. Unbelievable...but guess what...you are a step ahead of it all. That is why you WILL beat this and win the Olympics!!!

Onward...

Hugs and love.

Incredibly, it takes me almost five iterative visits to Dr. Three's office before I can get complete records. Each time, something is missing.

When I see the records, I am disgusted.

I read Dr. Four's colonoscopy report. Her pre-scope consult explicitly described me as a patient who "never had any diarrhea." But after she had seen a huge cancerous tumour, her scope report described me as having "a longstanding history of bloody diarrhea."

I post:

BETTER STILL

posted by Robin McGee, Monday, July 5, 2010, 9:45 PM

Hello All:

Today I went to my doctor's office for the third time to get my records...still things missing. When my family doctor came out for a patient and said hello, I found I could hardly look at him. It is clear to me that I need a new family doctor. I can barely be in that office, after all that happened, without feeling queasy; and with all the ongoing inadequacy around getting these records correctly, my sense of mistrust just mounts. It is not a good thing to distrust one's doctor or his staff. However, as a cancer patient, I will not be seeing a GP for years—the Cancer Centre takes over everything, so I have some time to start looking.

Today I felt better than ever. My radiation oncologist told me that the DNA destruction of the tumour from the inside starts after three weeks—it is three weeks tomorrow. Every tiny bit of evidence that the tumour is shrinking gives me hope—and physical relief, as it was truly painful. No amount of skin irritation can come close to that pain, so I do not mind the minor side effects I have had so far.

Tomorrow is the World Cup Semifinal! I am rooting for the Netherlands.

My mentor and colleague Joelle Caplan calls me. Joelle had been head of psychology at the local hospital prior to her retirement: she recruited me from Ontario nearly 16 years before. Concerned by the sick feeling I have about Dr. Three, she encourages me to approach other physician friends to help me find a new family doctor. Because I do not want to presume on those friendships, I am reluctant to ask my doctor friends for help to escape Doctor Three.

"The time for scruples is over," she advises. "Call your next-door-neighbours, Bruce McLeod and Lois Bowden—they are both emergency room doctors," she urges. "I promise you, they will *want to* help you with this."

Trepidatious, I call. To my relief, Bruce is immediately responsive. Bruce and Lois have been helping me in many concrete ways: he has mowed my lawn, she has raked it. Lois, a famously fabulous cook, has brought over several of her gourmet soups in respect of my miserable liquid diet. She once checked my PICC line when it seemed compromised.

"Leave this with me for a day," Bruce says. "I will find someone good for you."

I see his return email. I go weak with relief. Dr. Adam Good[1] is willing to help me. "He recognizes the situation for what it is," Bruce writes, "and realizes that the profession definitely cannot abandon you now, as I knew he would."

I post in relief:

---

1   Not his real name.

SO MUCH BETTER TODAY

posted by Robin McGee, Monday, July 19, 2010, 6:15 PM

Hello All:

Today I feel very well—really, really well.

Is it because I was able to eat some SALAD and grape dolmades at Opa's for lunch? (I was concerned that my *When Harry Met Sally* raptures over the food would disturb the other diners!)

Is it because I am so near the end of treatment?

Or is it because (and I know this is the true reason) that I am so, so relieved to learn that I have a new family doctor? Adam Good has kindly agreed to take us on. I really cannot express the feelings of utter relief and gratitude. Only now am I appreciating how much of a burden that issue was to me. I feel like my family and I can now be safe, that someone has my back, and that I can go on now. It is like I am free of that horrible medical past. Special, special thanks to Bruce McLeod for arranging that for me.

Darlene W < 7/19/2010 8:28 PM >

I am so glad you had a great day! I am also very happy for you that you have Adam as a doctor. He is our family doctor too. I really like him. He has been a great support over the years with a variety of little medical hiccups. He has a nurse practitioner that we see more and she is very good too. You are so right: it gives peace of mind to know you have a family doctor you feel you can trust.

Hope tomorrow is another good day for you.

Kym H < 7/20/2010 8:42 AM >

So very glad to hear all your positive news...the eating part IS exciting, and the end of this week will give you a break from the treatment (and all the driving). To finally have a new doctor, one you can trust, must be just so stress-relieving for all of you. I am SO happy for you!! This release of fear and anxiety over not having a family doc will help your healing in so many ways.

Hope this week's treatments go well...

Love ya!

Marilyn L < 7/19/2010 6:36 PM >

ADAM GOOD IS A GREAT GUY.

Feeling Better
posted by Marilyn C at Monday, July 19, 2010, 9:38 PM

Congratulations, Robin. I was hoping you'd get Adam. He is VERY thorough. I know some of his patients and they love him.

I had him at the Emergency Room once and he followed up with me later in the week! I've never had that happen.

So much better today
posted by Daphne K at Monday, July 19, 2010, 7:04 PM

You lift my spirit! I can picture you in *When Harry Met Sally* eating your salad. So glad you are feeling better. I know you have the strength and spirit to beat this demon. God Bless Bruce McLeod! So glad to know you have a new physician.

Cindy H < 7/21/2010 8:31 AM >

I just love getting all your messages...they are so inspiring. Sorry I have not been in touch recently, nor have I helped in any way. I wanted to help with the gardening, but I am SO not a gardener. However, I do look forward to actually seeing you in person. I cheer you on daily and my daughter and I are forever giving "high fives" for Robin whenever we receive an email. You are a survivor in the true sense of the word, in your honesty and in your spirit.

You are a fighter and there is NO WAY you are about to be beaten. We women do not give up easily, if ever!!!

You are so brave. Just everything that has come your way has made me admire and adore you more. Nothing prepares us Robin for what you have had to go through. I truly believe everything happens for a reason and you are going to bring changes and hope to the meaning of colorectal cancer, and maybe even to the medical profession. It takes someone with your wit and intelligence to do that. Adam Good is a wonderful physician. He is not our doctor (we have Dr. Phillips), but because he shares the same office, our daughter goes to him frequently for her weekly allergy shots when our doctor is away. Adam is her favorite!!!

I'm off to learn something (!), though you have been my teacher this summer.

Have a great day!

Joelle C < 7/21/2010 10:49 AM >

Oh how good to get validation from Bruce and Adam! And you know it makes people feel good to be able to feel a part of a remedy!

I am feeling so many positive vibes about you, Robin! So is Agnes. Glad our talk was helpful to you too, dear Robin!

....

My mind continually wanders back to Doctors One, Two, Three, and Four. I wonder how each of them reflects on my case. *Are they appalled or contrite? Do they examine themselves or their conduct at all? Do they understand the mistakes they had personally made or take any responsibility for them? Do they lay the blame at the feet of the other doctors involved, in the same way they each abdicated responsibility for intervention to the next doctor?* Perhaps they do not think of me at all, except to shrug it all away. Maybe it means nothing to them. Maybe they do not give me a second thought.

I consider the risks of complaining about them to the College of Physicians and Surgeons of Nova Scotia. There could be serious repercussions to such a step. If I start down that road, would the stamina required sap me of the precious energy I need for recovery? So many books warn cancer patients that they need to be forgiving and accepting. Dwelling on the mistakes of the past and nursing resentments could undermine my recovery. If I do not let go of the wrongdoing, perhaps I would condemn myself to death.

But you might die anyway, my conscience tells me. *And no one—no patient, no doctor—would be the wiser.*

I wonder if making a complaint would somehow jeopardize my cancer care. What if my cancer doctors learned of my complaint? Were doctors like cowboys—would they circle the wagon train and protect each other? Would they give me poorer care if they learned I had complained about some of their own?

And what about my own community? The health community in our region was small. Would local doctors turn against me, and would that jeopardize any future collaboration on behalf of my own patients, if I am ever able to return to work? Two of the four doctors were colleagues I had known well and worked with regularly—how could I take an action that would humiliate or harm them?

I lie awake at night, questions and doubts circling over my insomnia like vultures. I think about others who may have been mishandled as I had been. I have visions of the other patients who had waited 18 months for Dr. Four, and I wonder who else might die from such neglect.

What will happen if I do not speak out? Doctors One through Four would continue to practice with indifference. No one would learn from the mistakes. *If I must die from this cancer,* I think grimly, *can I really go to my grave knowing I could have done more to protect others?* Could I dignify my own suffering and probable death by wresting something positive out of it for the sake of vulnerable ordinary citizens?

I wonder if there is a restorative justice process by which I can get all four doctors into one room to have them debrief and discuss my case, just to learn from it.

I tentatively call the College of Physicians and Surgeons of Nova Scotia to inquire about the process. The assistant who takes my call is impatient. She seems annoyed by my question about whether the doctors in my case could be compelled to collectively participate in a case review. Exasperated, she tells me that this is not an option. My only course, she tells me, is to complain about each doctor individually. The fact that they were entwined in a complex case of miscommunication with each other is not relevant. She tersely detailed the various levels of paperwork that I would be required to produce.

When I hang up the phone from her, I know what I will do. Instead of discouraging me, the call inflames me.

So this is the first line of defence against assaults on the medical profession, I think with gritted teeth. *For once, that College is going to deal with someone with a voice.*

What if I had been someone else? What if I had been a shaky little old lady, a terrified young mother, or a wordless disabled man? A brusque reception like that would have made me give up on the spot. *Not this time*, I think. For all those citizens who do not have the strength or resources to speak out against poor medicine, I will speak out. And I will bring to bear all the capacity I possess to do so, cancer or no cancer.

I am suddenly, firmly determined to prepare the best-documented complaint CPSNS has ever seen. If there is anything PhDs in psychology are good at, it is documentation. We undergo years of graduate training making written arguments using judiciously referenced documents. *Just watch me*, I promise them.

Writing the complaints takes many weeks. I write a letter regarding each doctor, specifying in a bullet list the core of my complaints for each individual. I write a cover letter detailing the entire narrative. I reference what each doctor had written in their records and letters; I contrast their documentation with their actions and inactions. I photocopy all the records in my possession, carefully indexing them to points in my narrative. CPSNS had recently published a series of guidelines for the efficient and ethical practice of medicine. In the text of each lengthy response, I cite the many CPSNS guidelines that had been violated in my case: for example, in Nova Scotia, patients have a right to know about inordinate wait times, and doctors are obliged to help patients whose condition is worsening. I spend days preparing and revising pithy and articulate missives. Three friends, some with medical backgrounds, assist me with the wordsmithing. Responding to those letters requires much of me: incisive scholarship, medical literacy, and emotional restraint.

I write as I bleed. I write as I vomit. I write as I ache from my radiation burns and radiation colitis. I write as I wonder if I will live to see the outcome.

When my four complaint binders are ready, I compose a cover letter to CPSNS. After the opening paragraphs identify me and the doctors in question, I add a summary:

1 August 2010

Dear College of Physicians and Surgeons of Nova Scotia:

...I understand that I must submit a complaint for each doctor individually. I have submitted four separate binders. I have prepared a cover letter for each doctor outlining my complaints against each. However, I have included in each binder my entire story, as I believe this best illustrates their cumulative errors and mismanagement. Each binder includes identical appendices of the documentation I possess. The necessary forms and releases are included for each of the four binders. I request that the CPSNS treat these four complaints as one investigation.

I do not take this step lightly. I understand how serious and painful a process this is. I know that these doctors did not give me cancer. However, their errors greatly reduced my chances of survival. I was a highly active, physically fit professional when these events happened to me: if medical mismanagement like this can happen to me, it can happen to anyone. I sincerely hope that your review of my case might lead to changes that could protect other vulnerable Nova Scotians...For my suffering or possible death to have meaning, I want to prevent such disaster from befalling any other patient.

Andrew and I drive to Halifax to deliver the binders to the College offices. We know the next step: each doctor will be given four weeks to respond to my complaint in writing. I will then get a second opportunity to respond to them. Finally, each doctor will respond to my second letter. When the process is complete, the College will appoint an investigation committee to review all the submissions.

I hand the binders across the big reception desk in CPSNS's handsome glass-walled office. As I look up, I see their motto on the wall. "Excellence in Medical Regulation" is written underneath their title. As the door swings shut behind me, I wonder if they will live up to that maxim.

10

I AM WAITING IN THE CHEMOTHERAPY UNIT ON THE 11TH
floor of the Victoria General Hospital to have the 5FU bottle
changed. A solid woman in her 60s settles into the chair next to me
in the waiting room.

"My hair is just growing back in," she says, touching her greying
curls. "I have just finished my breast cancer treatments. My hair is
much better than the last time I had cancer."

I turn to her, curious. "You have been through this before?" I
ask, surprised by her cheerful demeanour. She looks exceptionally
well.

She smiles and shrugs. "I had stage IV ovarian cancer eight years
ago," she says simply.

I am gobsmacked.

"How...?" I stammer. *Isn't late-stage ovarian cancer always lethal?*
"How did you *do* that?" I manage to utter.

"It was in my lungs," she says amiably, ignoring my shock.
"But cancer did not know who it was dealing with." She grins. "I
did things. I made things happen. My son started a charitable
foundation that supported women with ovarian cancer among
other things, and I am very active in that. I also got involved in
the national organization, Ovarian Cancer Canada, co-chairing the
local Walk of Hope and serving on the board of directors. It gave me
a 'helper's high.' I went to church and connected with my community. I exercised. I read every book I could find about other cancer

survivors, looking for their reasons for success. I used visualization to picture Pac-Man gobbling up those cancer cells. I volunteered for research into the BRCA genes. I made damn sure I got the best treatment I could. And I did it all again for this cancer."

Called down the hall to my appointment, I cast my eyes back to her as I leave. As I climb into the big reclining chairs used for chemotherapy, I think about her. Although I have certainly heard terrible stories about those who die from cancer, I have also heard astonishing stories of those who survive it. Some people survive despite all odds. I think about those survivors I had actually met: a man who survived stage IV esophageal cancer that had spread to his lungs—he recovered completely and was a volunteer with the cancer society. A woman given only one month to live with a rare neuroendocrine cancer who had just returned from a hiking holiday in England four years later. A man told he had less than six months to live with stage IV lymphoma, still cancer-free ten years later. A fellow psychologist beat the same kind of pancreatic cancer that killed Patrick Swayze. I was astonished to learn that one of my own colleagues—a vibrantly powerful and healthy man—had survived stage IV multiple myeloma 22 years ago! It is one thing to read about survivors. It is another thing to meet them in the flesh.

My chemoradiation treatments are coming to an end. The day is fast arriving when I will be disconnected from the bottle and the daily radiation treatments will cease. As I approach the finale, my symptoms escalate. Vomiting and diarrhea set in. I try hard to follow the advice they have given me. Many hours are spent sitting in a sitz bath of plain warm water. I use the fan and the aloe vera to try to cool my increasingly hot and reddening skin.

ONE MORE DAY

posted by Robin McGee, Thursday, July 22, 2010, 5:30 PM

Hello All:

Today we had our last brace of doctor's appointments for a while. Only one more day—tomorrow is my last radiation appointment, and the PICC line is taken out and the chemo bottle is detached. I can't believe that this leg of the journey is almost over. When I look over my past comments and all your encouragements, I realize how long a road it really has been.

Today all the doctors were pleased by my apparent resiliency to the side effects of combined chemo/radiation. They are pleased with my skin. They still do not understand my blood results, but they want to give it three more weeks to see if my lymphocytes can bounce back.

During the last three days of radiation, they give what they call a "boost." The tumour is more specifically targeted. This often includes targeting more of the intestine than usual, giving me intermittent diarrhea, but that hopefully resolves sometime in the next two weeks.

I am really looking forward to the rest from the continuous driving to treatment. I have not had a normal bath, eaten a raw vegetable, cooked a full meal, had a drink of alcohol, been outside during the daytime, or exercised using my arms for six weeks. Sometime over the next month, I will be able to reclaim some of these things. What a blessing that will be!

FRANKENROBIN NO MORE
posted by Robin McGee, Friday, July 23, 2010, 4:30 PM

Hello Everyone:

ROBIN IS OFF THE BOTTLE!!!!

Today they removed my chemo bottle, and the PICC line that went inside me. I cannot express the relief at having my left arm back. Even to walk is easier. I have a bandage on it that I must wear for 2 days, but then I will be free to SWIM, SHOWER, and generally MOVE ABOUT! One of my first acts upon getting home was to book a massage therapy appointment for my left arm and shoulder—I have been carrying them awkwardly for six weeks, and my muscles have felt that constraint.

For some reason, our water has just gone off. Andrew thinks it is a local cessation. That is scary news to someone who needs a sitz bath every hour or so!

And I had my last radiation today. The techs and receptionists all cheered for me.

We also saw the dietician, who gave me direction on maintaining a low residue diet and slowly adding more variety.

So now comes a time when I can rest! It is like finishing a brutal final exam, like the last day of school, like hearing the ref whistle blow at the end of your most grueling game. I would drink to celebrate if the chemo had not killed my taste for it. Maybe lots of nice napping will substitute for wine?

NO BUTTERFLIES
posted by Robin McGee, Monday, July 26, 2010, 10:45 AM

Hello All:

I would love to tell you that I spent the weekend gamboling bottle-free through sunlit meadows alight with butterflies, but alas, the truth was not quite that way. I spent it between my bed and the toilet, struggling with symptoms so severe I had to miss the visitation and funeral for my friend Dana Patterson. I have had to call on all my psychology pain-reduction skills (think childbirth breathing) to get through the worst bits. For the sake of the squeamish, I won't elaborate.

This kind of suffering lasts a week—two at the most. As bad as it is, it is still better than when I started. I still have a partial bowel obstruction, which accounts for some of the pain. In six weeks or so, I won't have that anymore—the evil C will be cut out. Oddly, I look forward to that.

My big ambition today is to attempt a trip to the store. Wish me luck!

Tomorrow, Austin goes to his friend Isaac's cottage for a week (God bless the Berrys for this!), and on Wednesday Andrew and I will go to spend a few days alone at a cottage lent to us by our friend Stef Hurley. I am dearly looking forward to a change of scenery and some fresh air.

Welcome to midsummer!

Lesley H < 7/26/2010 12:40 PM >

Hi Robin—

I read with glee the ending of radiation and chemo for you, and then I read this. My heart is going out to you at the same time as you have become my absolute hero. You are an inspiration in perseverance; you have what it takes to run marathons, which is what this is. May you have moments of freedom from suffering and joy and bliss to carry you through the pain. May the cottage be a piece of heaven for you. You so deserve it.

....

I awake. Something is different. It is about 10 days since radiation ended. When I cast back the bedclothes, I see a livid burn covering my entire torso down to mid-thigh. Blisters are forming along my perianal area.

I call the clinic. Dr. Bahl allows a script for Flamazine, an antibiotic cream for second-degree burns. He knows what is coming.

I blossom in burns. I am bleeding from the burns in my rectum and the first third of my vagina. The pain is excruciating. I cannot walk for more than a few steps.

Andrew and I crawl away to a friend's cottage for a few rainy days. Hunched over the sitz bath in the tiny cottage washroom, I read Suzanne Collin's *The Hunger Games*. The story is both compelling and evocative. The main character is Katniss, a 17-year-old living in a post-apocalyptic world that has been divided into districts governed by a wealthy Capital. Each year, the corrupt Capital demands an entertainment: a boy and a girl from each district are selected to participate in the "Hunger Games," a televised arena in which the contestants must fight to the death. Katniss's story is a desperate and compelling story of survival as she faces her deadly competitors. As I read about her fighting to overcome burns, hunger, and savagery over weeks in the arena, I feel myself responding powerfully.

When I come home, I post:

HAMMOCK TIME

posted by Robin McGee, Sunday, August 1, 2010, 10:15 AM

Hello All:

I hope you are all enjoying the long weekend. Andrew and I were able to get away to that beach house. We could not go out much due to rain, but that was fine with us. I cannot do much anyway. My burns, which had been manageable first-degree burns, suddenly turned into second-degree burns (blisters and bleeding). I won't tell you where. I have a cream I can put on that helps to heal them, and that seems to be slowly working.

We laid around and watched movies. We watched the charming Disney movie *Up*. We cried our heads off at the part where the little old lady died before the little old man. I was sad because I really wanted to become a little old lady with my Andrew, and now I may not get that chance. So we cheered ourselves up with *Meet the Fockers*.

In happy news, I was able to have my first beer in months. Today I plan some hammock time, also a first. My dietician has allowed me to have two tablespoons of All Bran buds today. This amount will be slowly increased. So some things are looking like they can start to return to normal, or to a new normal. Yahoo!

Lisa P < 8/1/2010 4:39 PM >

You WILL become a little old lady, Robin. Remember...those statistics they quote include the non-believers too. This thing will not beat you. Believe in your mind and body. There is a lot more there in us than we give ourselves credit for. When it is kicking your ass (as it seems to be at the moment...I hope the cream is helping), you can kick its ass waayyyy harder! It won't be coming back to Robin's town any time soon!

Susan B < 8/1/2010 10:45 AM >

Oh Robin,

My heart skipped yet another beat when I read about your and Andrew's cry during Disney's *Up*. I am so happy that you have each other. I write this email with tears and continued hope for your complete recovery. I think of you and your family daily and pray for strength for you all.

I hope that you get to have another beer soon, that your burns feel better even sooner, and that your "new normal" is always manage-able no matter what that may happen to be.

I hope that you enjoy your day and hammock.

Rita V < 8/3/2010 9:29 AM >

Dear Robin

I have been thinking about you a lot, and after reading your note, I want to make sure that you are doing well. Sounds like the radia-tion burns are pretty painful and have increasingly become more raw and painful.

Robin, you are going to be an old little lady with your Andrew!!!!! I have a strong conviction that it will be so.

Is there anything that you need done? Let me know.

....

Dr. Bahl had warned us at the beginning of radiation: it can significantly damage the vagina. "Use it or lose it," he told us. He recommended that I check my vagina with my own fingers about two weeks after the end of radiation.

When I do, I am horrified.

Inside, the walls are webbed with adhesions. Thick ropes of scar tissue cross inside it like a spider web. *The walls are fusing together.* Terrified, I claw out the adhesions with my bare hands.

Panicked and sickened, I call the Cancer Centre. I also call a friend who had undergone internal pelvic radiation. "You need to demand some vaginal dilators," she tells me firmly. "Don't let them put you off."

"What the hell is a vaginal dilator?" I ask. I have never heard of such a thing.

"They look like test-tubes. Like a smooth plastic cylinder. They come in different sizes. You start with the smallest one and work up to the biggest one. You have to put them inside you for about 10 to 15 minutes."

"How often do you have to do that?"

"Everyday, once you get them. After a month you can back off to five days a week for six months."

I shudder at the thought. My internal flesh is so raw. "And after that?"

My friend laughs grimly. "According to the pamphlet," she says, "at least twice a week for the rest of your life."

I leave a message at the Cancer Centre, asking for dilators. But when I check my phone, I find a message saying that vaginal dilators are only given to women who have undergone internal radiation, not external pelvic radiation like me.

A cursory internet review teaches me that it is a standard of care in the United Kingdom for *every* woman who has undergone external radiation to receive dilators. I read to my mounting anxiety that there is a window of opportunity for dilator use, and that failure to use the dilators within the necessary time frame can result in permanent vaginal stenosis and destruction. Indeed, some women become medically unexaminable. I reflect with frustration and anger that I would not even know to ask for these dilators if I did not have a friend who was open about needing them during her own cancer treatments. How many women are so lucky? What is happening to other women out there?

I call the Centre back, this time insisting on speaking to my own radiation oncology nurse. Cara seems to hear the distress and anxiety in my voice. She assures me that she will give me a dilator set, leaving it at the front desk in a brown bag. Andrew will need to drive into Halifax to get it. I cannot help shivering.

....

The day has come for Ron's memorial service. His children and grandchildren will go to sea to launch the tiny wooden vessel Andrew has so carefully crafted.

THE VOYAGE OF THE *RON HURST*
posted by Robin McGee, Monday, August 9, 2010, 2:00 PM

Hello All:

Yesterday, we went to sea to launch the *Ron Hurst*, our memorial to Andrew's father, who died of cancer a month ago. There are a few photos on the Photo Gallery, which show her launch into the sea. She needed some significant last-minute modifications by Andrew to improve her seaworthiness, but she handled beautifully.

We went out past the harbour mouth, past McNab's Island, past Eastern Passage, to just abeam the belled red buoy near Devil's Island. Austin read the memorial poem, and we set her alight on the water. She slipped out of Andrew's hands like a minnow and darted off to sea. She took a comfortable tack out to sea with the tide, valiantly cresting the waves as she headed out to the open ocean. We watched her go away on her adventure, until she was lost from view.

Some of you may know that I have an undergraduate degree in English as well as psychology. So I found the ideal poem for the memorial: John Masefield's "Sea Fever." It was the perfect poem to describe Ron's life:

I must go down to the seas again,
to the lonely sea and the sky,
And all I ask is a tall ship
and a star to steer her by;
And the wheel's kick and the wind's song
and the white sail's shaking,
And a grey mist on the sea's face,
and a grey dawn breaking.

I must go down to the seas again,
for the call of the running tide
Is a wild call and a clear call
that may not be denied;
And all I ask is a windy day
with the white clouds flying,
And the flung spray and the blown spume,
and the sea-gulls crying.

I must go down to the seas again,
to the vagrant gypsy life,
To the gull's way and the whale's way
where the wind's like a whetted knife;
And all I ask is a merry yarn
from a laughing fellow rover,
And quiet sleep and a sweet dream
when the long trick's over.

....

ROBIN McGEE

Still shaken by the strange hemorrhage, the premature menopause, and the vaginal burns, we had asked Dr. Bahl for a referral to gynaecology. We have not heard anything in weeks. When we call Cara to find out what happened, her investigations reveal that the referral was redirected to local gynecology, and in that process it became lost.

Our wise Dr. Good anticipated this. "If that referral falls through somehow," he had said, "call my office and we will make one for you." I was delighted to hear that one of my options was Dr. Gillian Graves of the IWK Health Centre.

I had known Dr. Graves from the past. She had been one of the gynaecologists I had seen repeatedly during my secondary infertility treatments over a decade before. She is a mature woman, diminutive and wryly funny. I remembered how approachable she had been with me—we had often discussed books while she prepared me for those dreadful procedures. I also knew her to be a woman of tremendous integrity. A close friend of mine had gone into the dangerous condition ovarian hyperstimulation after an in vitro fertilization procedure. She spent three weeks in hospital near renal failure. Dr. Graves was not my friend's doctor—but nevertheless, she visited my friend in hospital every day. I learned that Dr. Graves had advocated on behalf of my friend, crossing swords with certain colleagues in the process.

When she received my referral from my new family physician, Dr. Graves scrambled to get me in before my cancer surgery. *Good on you, Girl*, I think gratefully. *Another example of how the truly professional doctor functions.*

Dr. Graves is as funny and warm as I remember her. I describe to her the brutal hot flashes I have developed since radiation. These are not moderate flashes—they are crushing, nauseating, I-need-to-sit–down experiences. The sensation of every capillary clenching down on itself is as excruciating as crunching one's teeth on ice, bruiting all over my ravaged body. Sleep, always elusive to a cancer patient, has become impossible. She nods with familiarity and understanding.

She examines me and affirms that my vaginal tissues have been significantly damaged by both radiation and the premature menopause into which the treatments have hurled me.

"You went from having the hormones of a 48-year-old to those of a 68-year old in two months, and that was on top of the radiation," she explains. To describe my stenosis, she humourously tells me that I am a "one-finger woman" and that I need to be a "two-finger woman" in order to be sexually functional. She supports the use of vaginal dilators, but she encourages me to consider getting a better "more fun" one from a sex shop. Once I am able again, she encourages us to use "natural methods" instead of the dilator to maintain my size. She offers to prescribe a vaginal suppository that would supply estrogen to the area. Once my treatments are over, she will recommend hormone replacement therapy.

"How long would I take the vaginal estrogen for?" I ask her from the examining table as she heads towards her desk.

"Until you are 85," she calls back.

I laugh. "That means you think I am going to make it until I am 85?"

She stops midway to her desk and turns around to face me. She is grinning her impish grin.

"*You* are going to make it," she says.

....

I am in the sex shop Venus Envy, on Barrington Street in downtown Halifax. I have never been in a store like this in my life. My friends Thea and Pam are with me, giggling. They shoulder me up to the cash register, where a woman with a nose ring and many tattoos waits for us to approach.

Blushing furiously, I awkwardly explain what I have come there for. To my relief, the staff person responds with understanding confidence. "We get lots of cancer patients here," she reassures me. "Come with me to the back."

The back wall is covered with dangling dildos in all states of realism. Furtively glancing at them in curiosity, I try to appear disinterested. *What is that? Is that one for real? Is that one moving?* I worry about knocking one off the wall by accident.

"This is what you need over here," says the staff. She lifts from the shelf a sedate, conventional-looking box. I blush again with relief at its apparent normalcy.

She pulls the device from the box. "This is called a Berman dilator," she continues. "It is plain and smooth, which is best for women with damaged tissues like yours. You don't want anything bumpy or with jagged edges. You don't want anything with moving parts. This one has graduated sizes to use as you get better." She pulls off the outer sheath, revealing the smaller sheath below. I am reminded of the Russian dolls that fit inside each other. "And it vibrates, which creates more blood flow to the area, and that can speed up the healing of damaged tissues..."

She turns it on and hands it to me. I take it gingerly. "We sell a lot of these," she says supportively, "and not just to cancer patients. Women in menopause and very young women sometimes need these too."

So I join other sisters, I think. I turn it off and put it back in its modest box. *God love us.*

11

THE RADIATION EVENT IS OVER. THE SURGERY EVENT MUST begin.

It has always been my way, when trying to wrestle with an issue, to think it through by integrating it with the great literature I have read. When trying to come to terms with the prospect of surgery, as well as the prospect of death, I turn to those writings.

In Shakespeare's *Measure for Measure*, Claudio faces his execution the next morning. Others try to persuade him that death is valiant, easy, and preferable. He responds:

> *Ay, but to die and go we know not where;*
> *To lie in cold obstruction, and to rot;*
> *This sensible warm motion to become*
> *A kneaded clod; and the delighted spirit*
> *To bathe in fiery floods or to reside*
> *In thrilling regions of thick-ribbed ice;*
> *To be imprison'd in the viewless winds,*
> *And blown with restless violence round about*
> *The pendant world; or to be worse than worst*
> *Of those that lawless and incertain thoughts*
> *Imagine howling! – 'tis too horrible*
> *The weariest and most loathed worldly life*
> *That age, ache, penury, and imprisonment*

Can lay on nature is a paradise
To what we fear of death. (2.1.116-29)

I read again the final scene in Hemmingway's *For Whom the Bell Tolls*. The protagonist is lying on the ground, awaiting the enemy soldiers who are coming up the hill towards him. He knows they will kill him when they do. He reaches down to touch the pine needles on the forest floor, aware that he is in the last minutes of his life.

One of my favourite novelists is the visionary and mercurial Fyodor Dostoevsky. When he was a young man, he was arrested for consorting with some student critics of the political regime. He was made to face a firing squad—but this was merely psychological torture: on the spot, his sentence was commuted to imprisonment and penal servitude in Siberia. The great writer was forever altered by this cruel experience. In his book *The Idiot*, the main character autobiographically describes his thoughts at the time of this event:

> A priest went about among them with a cross: and there was about five minutes of time left for him to live...He wished to put it to himself as quickly and clearly as possible, that here was he, a living, thinking man, and that in three minutes he would be nobody; or if somebody or something, then what and where? He thought he would decide this question once and for all in these last three minutes. A little way off there stood a church, and its gilded spire glittered in the sun. He remembered staring stubbornly at this spire, and at the rays of light sparkling from it. He could not tear his eyes from these rays of light; he got the idea that these rays were his new nature, and that in three minutes he would become one of them, amalgamated somehow with them.

In the same way, I am finding that my life is passing before my eyes. But in slow motion. My death is not immediately imminent, but nevertheless I am often seized by memories that arise out of my own impermanence. I suddenly and vividly remember the smell of the acorns on the playground of my elementary school, the heft of raising my toddler to my hip, the sight of snow on branches at dusk walking in the long blue shadows of an Ottawa twilight.

I read again the scene in which the battleship has sank in Monsarrat's *The Cruel Sea*. The survivors are clinging to the life raft in the North Atlantic. One is a young sailor with the first symptoms of venereal disease burning in his groin. He opens his mind and body to let the cold seawater cool him—but in so doing, he lets death in too.

I put down the book. *You must hang on*, I think. *But you must not let death in.*

I post:

APPROACHING SURGERY
posted by Robin McGee, Sunday, August 29, 2010, 6:00 PM

Hello All:

I hope everyone is enjoying the last true summer weekend. We got Austin's cool school clothes, and we saw *Twelfth Night* at Shakespeare by the Sea (a treat!). I was all set to visit my soccer team at their game tonight, but it was forfeit—too many players on the other team out relaxing! Who can blame them?

Some of you have asked how I feel about my approaching surgery. On Sept 14th, I will have my abdomen cut open vertically (a nice bisection with my pre-existing Caesarean scar) and my colorectal area exposed. The cancer will be cut out, and the two healthy ends outside the margins will be stapled together—a resection. To allow the tissue to heal, they will divert my digestion through my small intestine, so I will end up with a temporary ileostomy.

So how do I approach this? I reflect upon all the remarkable survival stories I have read—of people lost alone in the North or in the Amazon—who somehow make it back to safety after weeks of privation. I reflect on that hiker who, alone and with an arm crushed beneath a boulder, cut his own arm off with pocket knife and hiked back to civilization, elated to have saved his own life. Like anyone else who reads such stories, I wonder if I could have the courage to do what these men and women have done. Would I have what it takes to cut off my arm if it meant I would live? My surgery is no less intrinsic to my survival: I will die without it. What body part is one willing to live without if it means retaining your life? Those brave people had to pay a price to live, and surgery and disfigurement is my price. Unlike them, I will at least have the benefit of an expert surgeon and general anaesthetic!

So I approach surgery with acceptance and resolve, surrendering to the truth that it is my only choice if I want to stay with my family and friends—and, of course, I do.

Patricia M < 8/29/2010 8:19 PM >

Oh Robin:

You are certainly to be admired. A strong spirit. I admire you.

As one who has recently had major surgery (we will have to share scars some day), I thought I should tell you that I had a great sense of peace throughout the process. Maybe resignation! I cannot say I was ever terrified. I felt that God was with me and that I was in His hands and whatever happened would be his decision and it would be OK. Even the night before surgery, I just rolled over and went into a sound sleep. I guess that is peace. I was more curious when I went to the OR than scared. Maybe we have a strong family spirit and a strong faith.

So keep up your great spirit. I am and will continue to pray for you. Many of my friends are praying for you too.

P.S. It is OK to cry!

Debbie M < 8/30/2010 9:58 AM >

You are a brave woman. I think the following quote describes you well:

"The idea of warriorship is that the warrior should be sad and tender, and because of that, the warrior can be very brave as well. Without that heartfelt sadness, bravery is brittle, like a china cup." (Chogyam Trungpa Rinpoche, Founder of Shambhala Buddhism)

Kym H < 8/29/2010 10:34 AM >

So eloquently spoken. You are my hero and a true role model. Your words will cause all who read them to pause and reflect on the true nature of what's really the most important thing in life. And as I have learned over the years, it all comes down to the relationships one has with family, friends, colleagues, and the world at large.

Sarah H < 8/31/2010 11:08 AM >

My dear Robin,

You are so brave. We will hold you in our thoughts and prayers while you enter this next stage of treatment. You are loved by many. Hold on to that.

SURGEON VISIT
posted by Robin McGee, Wednesday, September 1, 2010, 4:30 PM

Hello All:

Today Andrew and I met with my surgeon. He said that from what he can see the tumour has shrunk by about 50% by the chemo-radiation treatment over the summer. He repeated the details and risks of the operation. He reminded me that he may open me up and find that I am at a far more advanced stage than was thought, despite any previous imaging. He told me that they would have to remove affected organs (ovaries, uterus) if those were invaded.

This part gave me a jolt of fear. Cancer that advanced would be considered incurable. I settled myself by reminding myself that what is, is. If I am in stage IV, I am. I, like all of us, am nailed to reality as Christ was nailed to the cross. I was reminded of a patient of my own, who, when asked by a relative if she was mad at me for diagnosing her child with Tourette syndrome, replied, "But he had Tourette anyway, whether she said so or not." So if I am in fact terminal, I am resolved to see it as my truth, my time.

In other news, I met with Human Resources from the School Board the other day. I do not have sufficient sick days to carry me through two chemos and two surgeries. I did not know this, but sick days must be used up continuously and consecutively to allow access to Long Term Disability. So their advice was that I take off the entire school year, as this was better for both me and them, rather than having me come back for a few weeks at a time and jeopardizing the LTD I will certainly require. This came as a great surprise to me. Those of you who know me know that I love to work, and the thought of not doing it for such a long time is, well, weird. But this also means that I will be entirely well by the time I get back to work...assuming of course that I do not snuff it before then!

Special greetings to all of you in education, who had to return to work today. I am thinking of you all like mad.

Roger and Joan < 9/1/2010 8:56 PM >

Dear Robin,

Please know how much you are loved by all the professionals I know—and by so many, many families and children you have dedicated your life to.

If we all love you, how much more does a compassionate God, who created you and knew you before you were born?

"To live is Christ and to die is gain" (St. Paul)—but we are all continuing to pray that God isn't finished with you yet and we can continue to celebrate your presence here.

Never forget that He also created the surgeon, inspired him to go into medicine, and has honed his skills over the years. God will be guiding the surgeon's hands while He holds you in the palm of His hand—and in our hearts.

May He continue to inspire you to these courageous messages—thank you for having the courage to "tell it like it is" so we can stand with you—in love and hope.

Marilyn C < 9/2/2010 10:15 AM >

Wise, I think, to look at your life and risk of advanced disease as you are. The energy that you would use up worrying about that could be used to fight the disease that is quite possibly in the process of being arrested. I am amazed, however, that you are able to be so rational in the wake of this evil disease. I would undoubtedly take the unwise route! :)

I do believe that we all come into this world with an assignment or, at the very least, an expiry date, and when it is up, it is up! I do not, as I keep saying, sense that yours is up.

Wise counsel as well, I think, to stay out of the germ-infested schools. I just visited all of the classrooms at my school and found several children missing already due to stomach flu. And how readily others were to volunteer the info that they, too, had the bug as recently as yesterday!!!

Enjoy the rest. Or write a book! (my dream)

Suzanne S < 9/3/2010 12:53 PM >

Your visit to the surgeon would frighten the strongest of people. It is encouraging to hear the tumour has shrunk to half the size. I'm sure your psychology background has been a great resource for you as you continue to face each step of your journey.

We will continue to focus on a positive outcome for your surgery.

I will continue to keep you in my prayers each day!

Beth R < 9/5/2010 10:47 AM >

I had wished that I could donate my sick days to you if there were some provision for doing so. Now I wonder if the LTD isn't the better route. From my recollection, it was nontaxable income and thus financially puts recipients in a better position.

I am hoping, along with all of your circle of caring friends and family, that the surgical findings are consistent with the imaging, with no surprises unless those of a positive nature.

It truly will be a very different year for you to not be rushing in a million directions to meet a million needs and instead being able to focus solely on the needs of you, Andrew, and Austin. This gift of time for healing, reflection, revisiting priorities, and pursuing dreams is well deserved. Perhaps you, Andrew, and Austin might be able to plan a special trip to take place during the later stages of your healing.

Thinking of you often, and wishing you a safe journey through surgery and beyond.

A ROOM FULL OF ROBINS

posted by Robin McGee, Thursday, September 9, 2010, 4:15 PM

Hello All:

There have been some more developments that have given me great relief. In fact, I think I could dissolve with relief. Austin will be staying with Glen Berry and family while I am in hospital during the schooldays. Glen's son Isaac is Austin's best friend. A lifelong friend, too. We have pictures of them crawling together. Although Austin wanted to convey to us that he was able to spend the 10 days at home alone, I could see the relief in his face when we told him we had made these arrangements. I am so glad to know that he will be looked after and has people around him during the difficult days ahead. God bless the Berrys!

I have invented a new psychological technique that I have been using on myself with good effect. (Psychologists among you may recognize a variant of the "Dissociative Table" technique here). Of late, I have had moments of real fear, sometimes blindsiding fear. To manage, I envision a room full of Robins. In the room, there is professional Robin, mother Robin, playful Robin, soccer Robin, literature-reading Robin, etc. The doorbell rings and outside is Fear Robin. The Robin who answers the door says, "Oh, it's you. You should come in." The other Robins get Fear Robin a stiff drink and tell her to sit down on the couch. I imagine them all interacting. Somehow, I find this imagery instantly calming. (Maybe because it reminds me vaguely of the funny sketch in Monty Python where Death shows up at the door after the partygoers have eaten the salmon mousse). Maybe once I am better, I could write this technique up for a journal or book! Maybe then I could introduce talk-show Robin!

Joelle C < 9/9/2010 6:36 PM >

You continue to amaze me. Add Courageous Robin to the room and give them all a hug from me!

Beth R < 9/9/2010 7:05 PM >

I love this, Robin! You absolutely should think of writing this up. Of course, if you then go the talk show route, you'll have to decide which Robin is going to get stage time!

Corena B < 9/9/2010 8:10 PM >

And also in the room with all the Robins, as Fear is invited in, is a bevy of strong women supporting all the Robins. We are caring for their needs as we are able to, allowing Fear to have a small space in the room, and acknowledging its presence and right to be there, but not allowing that Robin to control.

You are amazing! Love and strength to you!

Thea B < 9/9/2010 8:12 PM >

Do you think the calmness comes from the stiff drink? I'm assuming you actually pour yourself a scotch!

See you Saturday.

Linda G < 9/10/2010 9:42 AM >

Leave it to you, the therapist, to come up with a loving, supportive approach for yourself...you could indeed see this as a pilot study. It makes sense that it would be helpful. And again, think of all the different types of situations you'll have firsthand knowledge in how to handle...He will make you a better therapist!! You're in my prayers.

Tara S < 9/13/2010 11:28 AM >

I think you need to add Mentor Robin, who would be looking very wise and calm, and sci-fi/Tolkien Geek Robin to the group. The interactions would be extremely enjoyable to observe!

··········

It is the day before my surgery. I post:

BIG DAY TOMORROW
posted by Robin McGee, Monday, September 13, 2010, 9:15 AM

Hello All:

Well, tomorrow is the big day. I am looking forward to it. Today is the bowel prep, which is a significant chore, but I am "up" for that too. The biggest hardship is no food—clear liquid only today.

The surgery is scheduled for 7:30 am. I have to be at the hospital for 6 am, meaning we must leave here no later than 5 am. It is expected to last around five hours.

I hope to listen to my "successful surgery" visualization mp3 during the surgery. That visualization has me in the OR with the supportive presence of all those who wish me well. To all of you who are sending healing and supportive thoughts and prayers— send that energy along early tomorrow morning, and you will be with me.

Andrew will try to post something on the website tomorrow to let you know how things went. I will be out of communication reach for many days afterwards. I am not sure if I will be visitable at all. Even Austin won't see me until the weekend. Watch the website for updates from Andrew on my status for calls and visits.

My love to everyone.

Time to cross the Rubicon.

Heather R < 9/13/2010 9:46 AM >

Dear Robin,

God speed you through the long-distance run tomorrow. You will win the event as you understand and practice the positive thinking all Olympic athletes use!

You will be the focus of my yoga practice for the rest of this week.

"Namaste" (the light within me honours the light within you).

Sharon R < 9/13/2010 3:07 PM >

Robin, I have been a quiet supporter throughout the summer. However, I will focus my happiest, best, and loudest of wishes to you early tomorrow morning.

I have always had many things to thank you for as you worked with my students. Now I can add my thanks for your humbleness. You have helped me deal with something over the summer months; you have given me personal strength and confidence once more.

I will be thinking of you, great big wonderful thoughts.

Alison L < 9/13/2010 3:46 PM >

You will be in our prayers tonight, tomorrow, and ongoing days. We pray for the doctors to do a bang-up job; we pray for you to be relaxed, stress free, and heal well. God bless. Will Andrew be in the city or home? Would he like meals?

Claire W < 9/13/2010 7:49 PM >

Best of luck with everything tomorrow. Heather H and I are running on the dykes at 7 am, and we will think about you and talk about you and send positive sweaty thoughts your way the whole time! You are strong, Girl. You will do great…

Sherrie C < 9/13/2010 12:10 PM >

You will be surrounded by Ravens in thought and prayer!!

Linda G < 9/13/2010 9:38 AM >

You're in His hands...the best place to be!!

Rita V < 9/14/2010 10:09 AM >

My love to you Robin!!

I look forward to hearing from you and Andrew about the success of the surgery. I must say, over the course of your cancer journey, I have gotten to respect you so much more and there was loads of respect before. I also have learned more about you, your resilience, your strength, your positive outlook, etc. It seems that this journey has strengthened your bonds with everyone including me.

I'll talk to you soon.

Cindy H < 9/13/2010 9:47 PM >

We are thinking of you constantly. Stay focused and know we all care about you so much. And this surgery...it's all good! I feel the "Robin karma!!!"

Wanda C < 9/13/2010 5:33 PM >

My thoughts and prayers are with you and will continue to be throughout your successful surgery and recovery. You have been so open about what you have been going through and that has been a huge help to all of us dealing with similar situations with our families. I, as well as many others, will be watching the website for the latest updates. Sending positive vibes your way as always. Hugs to you, Andrew, and Austin.

Suzanne S < 9/13/2010 4:10 PM >

I'm glad to hear the day is finally here, and I wish you a successful surgery and a speedy recovery. If anyone has the tools to cope with this, it is definitely you. As I mentioned before, I have three friends who have come through colon cancer in the same stage as yours. I am happy to say that all three are now well. One of our closest friends is in his 12th year since diagnosis. I am praying for you each day and am optimistic that you will join my friends in beating this cancer. I'll say extra prayers for tomorrow's surgery.

Take care and stay positive.

Surgery
posted by Emily F at Monday, September 13, 2010, 9:32 PM

I have been thinking of you all morning and reciting the poem, *Invictus*, in my mind. I truly believe that you, like Nelson Mandela, are "unconquerable" because of your indomitable spirit. The treatments may sap your energy for a bit, but they cannot take away your courage and inner strength.

Dolan and I will be thinking about you tomorrow as you experience the next phase of your treatment. We will be adding our prayers and hopes for positive outcomes to those of your numerous friends and supporters. You are a very resilient woman and a fierce competitor who deserves to win this battle. God Bless You.

Cheering Robin On
posted by Marilyn C at Monday, September 13, 2010, 12:21 PM

Hi all,

I just posted a suggestion on the message board section for a group cheer at 7:30 am tomorrow.

Joan B < 9/13/2010 10:35 PM >

LOVE LOVE LOVE AND LOTS OF PRAYERS FOR YOU!!

What an inspiration you are to all of us reading your emails. I found a photo of you and put it up front and centre on my bulletin board.

I think of you *so much*. I will hold up you and Andrew and Austin to God in prayer all day tomorrow.

Beth R < 9/13/2010 8:17 PM >

I second Margie's feeling that you have so many friends, family, acquaintances, and even those who barely know you sending love, prayer, well wishes, and other positive energy, that the energy field could literally cradle and support you.

May all go smoothly and gently tomorrow on your body and spirit. Wishing you, Andrew, and Austin many sunny days and years to come.

And messages poured in from the schools and teachers I had worked with for years:

Judy K < 9/13/2010 10:03 AM >

All our love and prayers go with you from Glooscap School.

Jude

Paula M < 9/13/2010 7:54 PM >

Dear Robin!

Our collective thoughts, prayers, and best wishes are with you. We will be thinking of you often tomorrow.

Love, the staff of Somerset School!

David C < 9/13/2010 11:59 AM >

Hi Robin...wishing you all the best tomorrow. Your friends from Three Mile Plains School are with you!!!!

David and staff.

Darlene W < 9/13/2010 8:05 PM >

Definitely sending lots of positive, happy thoughts your way for tomorrow and the days ahead!!!! I'll anxiously wait to hear reports from your husband.

GO ROBIN!!!!

Susan B < 9/14/2010 6:44 AM >

Well, this is it! The big day is here for you, and as I embark on another day at AEES school, you are at the forefront of my thoughts and prayers. Your strength and the love of family and friends will hopefully be ever present for you throughout your day today. What a marathoner you are...Definitely one of the best class acts that I have had the privilege to know.

God Bless and Safe Travels.

Messages arrive from other cancer survivors:

Daphne M < 9/13/2010 10:08 AM >

Hi Robin,

I'm sending all my good thoughts out to you today, tomorrow, next day, and so on. I know how nerve-racking this day is. You should know, though, that from the minute you check in—early in the morning (I think I was there by 5:30 with my own pillow)—the staff is absolutely great (and fast) and you will be looked after every step of the way. That alone took so much of the anxiety away. And when you wake up to the good news you'll get, then things are well on their way! You'll have plenty of time to sleep and rest your body and not think of anything other than recuperating, so take advantage of that, Girl! And don't be a hero by not asking for pain meds like I did. :)

So to our "Well Robin," be prepared to flap those wings to a smooth and quick recovery! You'll have many kind thoughts going out to you tomorrow so be prepared to be lambasted by them, OK?

Take care, Well Robin...

Lady D

12

LOOKING GOOD!

posted by Andrew Hurst, Tuesday, September 14, 2010, 6:30 PM

HEADLINES:
Surgery Goes Well!
No Extra Cancer Found!
Robin is Looking Good!

DETAILS:

I (Andrew) met with Dr. McIntyre at about 11:45 as he came out of Robin's surgery. He was pleased with the process and results. The tumour, although "very large," appeared to be self-contained, was "easy to get at, and was easy to remove." Other than some enlarged lymph glands in the area that he said were "hard and odd looking but did not look cancerous," he saw nothing else worth taking out. The results for the lymph and "margin" samples will not be available for six to seven weeks, but he says that he's confident that they are good and even if they are not, the chemo process would be the same.

I didn't get to see Robin until about 4:30 and she was asleep until a nurse woke her around 5. I explained Dr. M's good news to her and her face (which was already looking pretty healthy) developed a strong but quiet glow. She was so happy to finally have the cancer out of her! I wish I had thought to bring a camera! Even in her heavily drugged state, she was lucid and inspired enough to refer to a quote she had read this summer by Churchill when he had just learned that the Americans had finally entered WW2 – something to the effect of "Tonight I will sleep the deep and comforted sleep of the saved." Then she started drifting off again. (I might just have some of that sleep myself tonight.)

Tomorrow, they say she may feel more pain as the freezing and general anesthetic will be worn off (she chose not to have an epidural), but they expect to have her up and walking. There is no Wi-Fi in the room, so I will have to continue to report for awhile. Thank you all for your thoughts and prayers.

Andrew

....

I am falling
My mind bears down upon itself, closing off.
I am falling
My percipience extends only a few minutes ahead, to the next visit by the nurse, to the cast of sunlight through the darkened windows. And throughout all I hear the desolate mechanical throbbing of the intravenous machine, mournfully measuring the minutes of suffering. The antiseptic smell of the hospital cuts through my nose like an acrid smoke.
I am feral
Opiate-induced hallucinations infiltrate perception. I see large insects. I watch as the shadows on faces deepen suddenly and grotesquely, making every visage vampiric.
I am in pain
Skewered by pain, clubbed by pain. *A bear is chewing through my hip.* Severed by the surgery, my abdominal muscles are no longer able to support my back. Pain becomes detachment, a numbness

that swells and bursts open like a poisonous flower. Nausea swims around and around.

The Victoria General Hospital is a very old building. It dates from 1948. The halls are very narrow, and with the equipment needs of the GI ward, very crowded. The pipes are so old that the water has been declared undrinkable. Private rooms are not available, as they are reserved for the immune-suppressed. Typically, there are four patients to a room. Although the staff do their best to avoid mixed rooms, often men and women are placed in the same room.

I am unprepared for the pain I see in others. I watch my fellow patients scream and writhe. I hear the wails of the lost and demented. I hear the midnight weeping of the very afraid.

At night, the loneliness of the hospital descends. The woman in the bed next to me is dying of liver cancer. She screams, paces, calls people on her cell, and watches TV at all hours of the night. I wear my headphones to try to block her out. I am listening to an audio-book of *The Secret Garden*—a book about children who discover the healing power of a garden that they tend. The story's images of greenery and life emerging from a springtime soil seem impossibly distant.

I am enduring, enduring, enduring

Over days, I surface and resurface. My mind and perception widens incrementally. I feel marginally better. They have provided me with a button that would deliver painkiller to a fixed amount. Initially concerned that my respiration was too slow on the night after my surgery, they had cut me to half the typical dose. But an observant anaesthetist was watching the rate of my button presses; through that method, she discovered that I was in great pain. She tells me that I have had 148 unmet painkiller requests during the past 24 hours—nearly five times what it should have been. She doubles the dose of the medication delivered with each button press. My unmet requests drop to the typical 40 a day.

Underneath my blankets, I check my body. Down the centre of my torso, the main incision is a train track of flesh and staples from pubic bone to above my navel. On the left of my abdomen, my new stoma is visible through a clear plastic appliance. Fashioned from a loop of small intestine, it looks like a pink and glistening circular nub. A tiny orifice has been cut in it to allow digestion to pass out. The nurses who observe it as they care for me comment on how "cute" it is and how perfectly it has been constructed.

Dr. McIntyre has been away for several days. He comes to see me near the end of my stay, accompanied by a serious-looking resident. Examining my abdomen, he is pleased with the status of the incision and the stoma.

"This woman," he explains to the resident, "has had a curative resection of a stage III node-positive rectal cancer. This means that her chances of survival have gone from 30% to 50%. She must undergo adjuvant chemotherapy as her next step, which might increase her chances of survival by a few percentage points. Because she was thin, her surgery was easier to do. We were able to get in easily and manage the resection easily."

So my life of physical fitness has not been a waste of time after all, I reflect.

He tells me the next steps: he will review me in a month, around the time my adjuvant chemotherapy must begin. Once I have recovered from chemotherapy, he will reverse the ostomy—that is, sew the orifice on the stoma shut and push the little lump of small intestine back where it belongs.

The two of them sweep out of the room before I can croak my thanks to him for saving my life.

....

Andrew, Austin, and many RCO members come to visit. Austin has brought me a homemade card. It is a colour recreation of the children's book *Guess How Much I Love You,* in which a mother and baby rabbit describe their mutual love as distances.

Austin has written:

> I found this book when I was upstairs looking through the Austin Box and immediately thought back to when you used to read this to me as a child.

I also found the script to the play I was in, and remembered how you convinced me into doing it, even though I didn't want to, and all the fun I had doing it in the end.

I found my middle school graduation certificate and thought of how you helped me through those three tough years.

I even found the prop for my Grade 3 science project you helped me take all the way to the science fair.

I really want to thank you for helping me through my entire life and I'll be happy to help you through the hardest year of yours any way I can.

Love from all the way to the moon and back,

Austin

I place his card on my bedside table, stealing encouraging glances at it as the hours stretch into days.

I am so helpless. I used to be the strong parent who did things for my family. Now I can do nothing. But at the same time, I glimpse a new horizon. We are all changing. My teenager has reached within his taciturn persona to share his love. My exhausted husband holds my hand at my bedside. My friends appear with gifts, humorous and kindly. Supportive messages pour in to Andrew from RCO. I am damaged, but I am emerging from the shell of pain as from a chrysalis. The tumour is gone. I can start over.

Andrew brings me home. My mind is still reeling from the suffering I experienced and witnessed. I am tentative as I move. My ears ring continuously, echoing from the cacophony of the hospital.

I sit carefully on my own bed. I watch as the golden light of a fall afternoon steals across the room to where I sit, stealthily retreating as the blue silence descends. My body and mind feel purple, like a bruise.

I am haunted

....

Two days pass. I shiver, cold with pain. My incision holds me down, pinioning me to the couch. I try to take in movies through a fog of headache and nausea.

A nurse from The Victorian Order of Nurses (VON) comes to check my incision each day. One experienced nurse notices how puffy one side of my abdomen seems to be. It looks like it is straining against my staples.

"I don't think those staples are ready to be removed," she says. There is too much swelling to the area. I think you should let your family doctor know that."

When I call Adam Good's office to report her concern, he tells me he will come by my house that evening. Dr. Good still makes house calls.

He is pleased with my mobility, but agrees we should wait on the staple removal. When I describe the feeling of pressure and discomfort I have, he looks concerned. I have been home from hospital only three days.

I wake up that night in agony. *Something is very wrong.*

13

By the morning, I am vomiting forcefully.

My VON arrives. Camille listens concernedly to my account of my vomiting. She notices a bulge above the stoma. When she changes the appliance that covers my ileostomy, she sees that the stoma is not moving. She records that nothing has come out of it since the night before.

She sits on the foot of my bed where I lie sweltering with pain.

"I am *not leaving* here until we speak to your family doctor," she says firmly. "I think you could be in obstruction—something is blocking your small intestine. Who is your family doctor? Give me your cell phone and I will call him myself."

Adam Good's office is closed on Fridays. She calls him on his personal cell phone. He tells her he will contact Dr. McIntyre for directions and then come directly to my house.

I marvel once again at the integrity of some health professionals. All four of my pre-diagnosis doctors seemed to sleep through my increasingly desperate presentation. But Camille and Dr. Good were the very opposite—vigilant, responsive, focused. Camille was refusing to leave until my crisis was over, despite the pressure of all her other patients and responsibilities. And here was Adam Good, coming to my house on his day off. *How was it that I could experience the very worst of health care, and then the very best?*

Dr. Good calls. He has reached Dr. McIntyre. My surgeon has recommended that I try warm fluids for a few hours; however, if I vomit again, he wants me in the ER.

I spend the day on the couch. I do not feel nausea—it is beyond that. I feel smashed, staggered, crushed. It is like being submersed in a bath with waters made of oppression.

Dr. Good arrives in the afternoon. I am sitting on the side of my bed, trembling. Adam explains what Dr. McIntyre had described to him: that an injured small intestine can crimp over on itself, like a kink in a garden hose. The hose can unsnarl if it is relieved of pressure—which often means hospitalization, with intravenous fluids and a nasogastric (NG) tube.

"Patients sometimes have an instinct for these things," Adam says. "I wonder if your feelings of pain and pressure was a signal of potential obstruction."

While he is talking, I get up and march to the ensuite, where I vomit green bile forcefully and repeatedly.

"I think I am in obstruction," I call wetly to him.

When I sit back down gingerly on the bed, Dr. Good sinks down to sit beside me.

"You need to go the ER," he says. "Right now."

Andrew grabs the bag he had prepared for me.

"One other question," Adam says. "I noticed something the other day. When Andrew was in my office and I asked if he would consider Dr. Four as an endoscopist, I saw him wince. Do you have a negative history with Dr. Four?"

Andrew and I exchange glances.

"You are very perceptive," I say carefully. "She was one of the four who ignored my cancer symptoms, and I have a complaint to the College of Physicians and Surgeons against her. I also have a letter from the College saying that it does not want me to have any contact with her."

Dr. Good pats me on the shoulder reassuringly. "Because I had a feeling about that, I checked the call schedule, and I saw that she is the surgeon on call for tonight."

"I cannot see her," I groan. "Can't they make some other arrangement?"

"I will call ahead to make sure that the ER doctor there knows you are coming and about this situation," he says. "I don't want you to worry about seeing her—things are stressful enough for you as an emergency patient without that prospect hanging over your head. Now remember, if you are in crisis and bleeding to death, you may *have* to see her."

Despite my pain, I shake my head scornfully. *If I was in crisis and bleeding to death, would Doctor Four find some way to speed me on my way?* Her College problems would vanish with me. What was the old joke? *Doctors bury their mistakes.*

"I cannot see her for her own protection as well as mine," I say. "We could never trust anything she did or said in this situation. If things went badly, it would make things very sticky for both of us."

Adam assures us that he will do his best to take care of it.

Andrew and I are at Valley Regional Hospital in minutes, and I am in one of the Emergency Room bays within the half hour.

A spare, dark-haired ER doctor enters.

"Timing is everything," he announces. "I understand you cannot see Dr. Four, but she is the surgeon on call for tonight. I have a plan to work around that. We will take an X-ray, and if a surgeon's opinion is required, I will see to it that you are taken by ambulance to Halifax."

I am instantly relieved by his friendly and frank manner. I watch him carefully for signs of irritation. He seems to have no rancour at all over the situation. *Is that a twinkle of respect in his eye?* I bless him inwardly for addressing the Dr. Four issue right away. Perhaps he understood that any patient in my circumstances would dread encountering a nemesis. Maybe he understood that any patient might fear that the ER doctors would close ranks around her. Whatever the reason, through the haze of my pain, I feel grateful to be so promptly unburdened of the dread of encountering Dr. Four.

Having an NG tube forced down one's throat is one of the most unenviable experiences in medicine: unlovely for the patient, but also for the administering staff. I can see that the two nurses are working to suppress their own gag reflex as they force the tube down my nose and into my stomach.

I vomit and vomit. The ER doctor puts a steadying hand on my shoulder as I heave repeatedly.

They guide me to the X-ray room. The X-ray technician is gentle and softspoken. "I have a strong family risk for your kind of cancer," he says as he positions me. "I could end up like you at any moment." I nod at him gratefully. It was not the first time that a health professional with a family history of cancer would share that with me to bridge the gap between us. *Health care is not divided into the vulnerable and the invulnerable,* I think. *We are all vulnerable.*

I am back in the emergency bay. Andrew is with me. He looks green.

The ER doctor enters. "The X-ray shows a distortion of your small intestine, which may be an obstruction," he says. "It is a good thing that you are such an efficient vomiter—your system is trying to unburden itself to take the pressure off. But this is something that requires a surgeon's opinion, so I will arrange for the ambulance now."

As I am being wheeled out to the ambulance, one of the nurses checks the clipboard at my feet.

"Aha!" she crows as she reads it. "Just as I thought. You have Adam Good as a family doctor! He has written 'rule out obstruction'—what a great doctor! He is always right."

My head is swimming with the Ativan they have given me. The pain is like having a pump inside me that is inflating, inflating, inflating my intestines. My internal organs are screaming at me that they are about to explode.

I bounce about as the ambulance drives the bumpy roads to Halifax. *I am safe from Dr. Four,* I think, *but now far away again from my friends and family.* I knew that poor exhausted Andrew was behind the ambulance, driving into his own dark night.

They take me to the Halifax Infirmary. I wait in the hallway outside the ER for what seems like hours, then wait longer in an ER bay. I continue to vomit efficiently.

A crowd of medical students gathers around me. The resident who leads them is unpleasant and rough. Without ceremony or preparation, he forces the NG tube further down my throat. "This is all your fault," he growls at me. "You must have eaten something wrong."

Finally, in the very small hours of the morning, I am wheeled up to the quiet of the orthopaedic ward. I am attached with many tubes to the relevant machines. A kindly nurse comes to sit by me. She has a questionnaire to read to me.

"Is your social support not good, good, or very good?" she asks, her pen hovering.

I think warmly about the RCO community, counting down the many names in my mind. "My social support is very good," I say at last. "Write that down."

"Do you consider yourself to be experiencing high stress, moderate stress, low stress, or no stress at all?" she reads.

Even through my drugged haze, I burst out laughing.

"Put me down as moderately stressed," I say, when my hilarity had fallen to a chuckle.

....

The care I receive in the Halifax Infirmary is excellent. The nurses are talkative, attentive, and supportive of one another. They are delighted with me, as unlike the majority of their patients, I can access the toilet on my own. They sympathize regarding the painful NG tube, describing how they loathe inserting them. I watch with admiration their Herculean care of the demented elderly woman with the broken arm who shares my room, who frequently attacks them when they try to assess her. The room itself is clean and spacious. TV is available, which makes the hours pass more easily.

A CT scan of the abdomen confirms it: an obstruction. A surgeon who looks like a high-school student tells me I will be there at least six days. The accumulation of bile will be pumped out of me, and I will exist only on intravenous fluids. Relieved of pressure, the intestine would likely unkink on its own. If not, surgery is a final option.

The worst of the experience is the NG tube. It presses against the back of my throat all day, and all night. To control the retching that results from a full appreciation of its presence, I bend my mind to imagine it as a sore throat.

The strenuousness of my vomiting has pulled apart my incision in places, popping some of the staples. Dr. McIntyre's perfect incision is now askew. It looks like the tire tracks left behind by a demented driver who has spun off the road.

On my last day, they take out the NG tube. A caring medical student removes the remaining staples from my cancer surgery.

When they leave me alone in the room, I sit up in bed, trembling. Tears come unbidden. As I take my first free breaths without the tube, I feel only gratitude. My setback is over. However, I am warned that another obstruction could occur at any time.

I come home again, weak, shaken, and vulnerable.

RECALLED TO LIFE
posted by Robin McGee, Thursday, September 30, 2010, 2:30 PM

Hello RCO:

I am finally feeling up to a post. There is so much to tell you all that I am not sure where to start.

First, the surgery. They whisked me in before I could write "Out, Vile Jelly!" (from *King Lear*) on my stomach to amuse the surgery staff. Afterwards, the surgeon told me that he gave me what he considers a "curable resection"—meaning that he got everything visible. He told me that certain nearby lymph nodes were calcified and did not look cancerous to him, but these still have a 50% chance of being cancer. Only pathology results will tell us. He told me that by virtue of the surgery, my chances of being alive in five years have increased from 30% to 50%.

Second, the VG. Think of a WW1 field hospital. People screaming, nurses overworked, constant noise and confusion.

Third, homecoming. I was doing well and was so grateful for the peace and quiet.

Fourth, the obstruction. I woke up in extreme pain in the wee hours of Thursday, and by Friday I was vomiting violently. My new and wonderful family doctor Adam Good made a house call and saw me in action, so to speak. He arranged for me to get to the ER and even called ahead to ensure they knew not to pair me with Doctor Four, the general surgeon in my horrible assessment story. As luck would have it, she was the surgeon on call that night.

The first ER doctor told me I was an "efficient vomiter"—a good thing when you need to get fluid out of an overwhelmed system. I demonstrated my skill for him several times! I thought I should add "efficiently vomiting Robin" to the list of Robins in my room.

Because an X-ray revealed a potential kink in my small intestine, a surgeon's opinion was required. So they sent me by ambulance to the QEII. I ended up in the orthopaedic ward, with a nasal gastric tube and IV fluids. The QEII environment and nursing care were excellent. Nevertheless, the experience was exhausting. The stamina required to endure that tube for days would make a marathoner weep. When I came home at last, I felt like a baby seal that had been clubbed.

My first night home was touch and go. The VON made an emergency 1 am visit at my request. She helped me fix up my appliance, which was burning me. She recommended I go back to the ER. I just could not face that prospect, so I tried to sleep, deciding to evaluate in the morning.

I made the right choice. The cramping had settled by morning, and now food seems to be going through me without incident. Last night, I had my first solid sleep in 2 weeks.

I am still tired, but not as devastated as I was. I am now up for calls, visits, and emails.

Colleen R < 10/1/2010 9:28 AM >

Robin,

To think of what you have been going through almost makes me weep. But then I read your sense of humour and feel your energy through your writing, and it makes me smile.

When my husband had his back surgery, he ended up with an obstruction. He was in severe pain and vomited (efficiently, I believe!!!!) for a day before they realized what was going on. He also had some allergic reactions to painkillers, so that's what they thought was happening. When I finally FORCEFULLY pointed out that he also had not used the washroom in two days, they decided an ultrasound might be helpful—thus the discovery of the obstruction. He had the NG tube too.

Anyway, I tell you that just so you know that I have some kind-of second-hand experience of the awfulness of it. I'm sure you and Philip (my partner) could have long discussions about it. He also amazingly maintained his humour throughout it all, once the vomiting and pain lessened. Also, let Andrew know I kind of understand what he has been going through. Phil was in the hospital for two weeks with a variety of complications, and I was so exhausted after it all, I barely knew my own name. Being the supporting person is an incredible role to take on, and it sounds like he has been doing a fantastic job. I truly appreciated all the updates he kept sending.

You have an incredibly strong spirit. I will continue, as many of us are, to send healing thoughts your way. And thoughts of peaceful sleeps, good meals, and laughter.

Daphne M < 10/1/2010 9:41 AM >

So now my Well Robin is shifting into Resilient Robin...what's next? Wow Robin, methinks!

Dear Robin, your adventures have been so challenging and I can only imagine how overwhelming this recent downswing (though now on the upswing) has been since your good news surgery. I think your friends have been waiting with bated breath for the next piece of news from Andrew these past few weeks. (Yes, and his emails, too, were quite entertaining).

Not that I can appreciate your pain with the "kink," but my brother-in-law suffers from obstructions that land him in the hospital for periods of time and there is nothing to be done but wait it out. He experiences tremendous pain and he is the type of outdoors guy who normally could withstand some discomfort, but he also has a lot of scar tissue left over from a couple of colostomies—both since reversed—that cause these obstructions. But neither does he maintain a good diet and his doctors have told him that this is the bulk of problem!

Regardless, I am very happy that you are on the road to recovery and in the comforts of your home and family. I hope you are able to get out in the sunshine and just let yourself lean back and close your eyes and know that you are through the worst of it.

Thinking of you...all the time...

Lady D

Darlene W < 9/30/2010 8:05 PM >

SO GOOD TO HEAR FROM YOU!!!!!!!! Andrew did a great job on your behalf. You two make a great team! I really don't know much about you or your family, though I am glad I do now. Wish it was under different circumstances.

I just wanted to say "Happy Birthday" for tomorrow (Oct.1). I'm sending TONS of warm and happy thoughts for you enjoying your day and being home.

Patricia < 9/30/2010 6:42 PM >

Dearest Rawbean!

I'm SOOOO glad you are home again and doing well! Thanks for explaining about the VG—I didn't understand why you wanted to avoid going back there.

I think it's good to be an efficient vomiter! To encourage myself when I have stomach flu, I always think of Hagrid's (from *Harry Potter*) philosophical words to Ron after the slug-eating spell goes wrong..."Better out than in."

Stefani H < 9/30/2010 3:32 PM >

She's back with flare and wit to boot.

I will throw in a meal in a basket for your family to consume at their readiness in our absence ('cause that's what I do)—so let me know what foods you can do and might be craving, my little triathlon psychologist—or what might help to feed those boys.

Valorie R < 9/30/2010 6:39 PM >

God bless you as you soldier on...although there are times you feel as if you can't go on—you continue and take one step at a time. I learned a valuable lesson about cancer: life is just a series of moments strung together, so live each moment as though there will be no more.

Grace M < 9/30/2010 5:23 PM >

I am so glad to hear that you are settled at home and feeling better.

You are very lucky to have Adam Good as your doctor. He came to your rescue when you needed him. It is so special that he made a house call to see you "in action!"

During the past few months, I think that you have jumped through the rings in Robin's Cancer Olympics—Bravo, dear Robin!

Have another good sleep tonight!

Diane H < 9/30/2010 6:35 PM >

Wishing you well. Your marathon continues and I love reading your entries (and Andrew's—he has a very different sense of humour from you). I can almost picture those words on your belly...too bad you couldn't do that!! Always thinking about you.

Peter M < 9/30/2010 3:27 PM >

Hi Robin:

I have been a silent but very interested (and concerned) observer/ reader of Andrew's and your updates. Please know my silence is not an indication of not thinking about you very often. I have been sending whatever positive energy a sceptical atheist can send.

Take care and I look forward to a long string of consistently encouraging updates on your improving health and comfort.

I can empathize with you to some extent. (Have you seen the movie *The Bucket List*? There is an interesting scene with Jack Nicholson being sick due to his chemo looking in the mirror—as dishevelled as only he can look—saying, "Some lucky bastard somewhere is having a heart attack").

Kym H < 9/29/2010 3:25 PM >

Oh Robin, what a week you have had!! The "efficiently-vomiting Robin" might come in handy when you get back to work, especially if you are consulting with a stubborn, obstinate person who won't listen to reason!!

IN PRAISE OF ANDREW

posted by Robin McGee, Sunday, October 3, 2010, 3:00 PM

Hello RCO:

I have had a chance to read over all the posts by Andrew, done while I was debilitated, and your kind and encouraging responses to him. He truly deserves all your praise and support. It is astounding what he has been through personally this year—nursing his dying father, moving through his death, and now caring for me through my similar struggles. Through it all, he continues to do much work around the house (his therapy—yay!!) His offbeat sense of humour keeps us in regular stitches. He wrote you about my face glowing as he gave me the news that the surgery had gotten all the cancer. From my angle on the bed, I saw his face alight with the same softened warmth with which he said our wedding vows 20 years ago (that is, when he wasn't giggling through them). Andrew truly has embodied the "in sickness and in health" part of that vow.

Each day I have been home, I have felt a little more well. I still have episodes of considerable pain, but it passes and I am functioning. I try to take a 30-minute walk each day. I lie down each afternoon, sometimes napping. I am watching lots of great classic movies on the Turner Movie Channel. I have learned that another obstruction could hit at any time, so I am grateful for each day that goes by without one.

Patricia B < 10/3/2010 5:37 PM >

You both got a keeper! I think you have learned how truly lucky you are to have found each other. Your love inspires me...

Debbie M < 10/3/2010 10:19 PM >

Yes, Andrew is the greatest, and I'm proud I have told him a few times now how awesome he is. He is setting the standard for spousal care very high!

Kym H < 10/2/2010 10:26 PM >

I agree with your evaluation of your Andrew: he IS a prince
and I am amazed by his enduring attentiveness and caring for
you. I came home and told Allen how wonderful Andrew is and
exclaimed how he waited on all of us Friday night when we had
our fish and chip dinner. I enjoyed his posts while you were in
hospital and I think the two of you should collaborate and write a
book about this experience. You both have a gift for expressing
yourselves with great wit and insight. A bestseller for sure!!

Hope you get the lasagna today that we left on the doorstep.

HAPPY BIRTHDAY TO ME
posted by Robin McGee, Friday, October 1, 2010, 2:30 PM

Hello All:

Well, today is my birthday. I am 49. I can think of better ways to
spend it than nursing myself, but at least I am still around to do
that. During my most recent hospitalization, one of the nurses
told me she was shocked to see my true age on my chart—she
thought I was in my early thirties! I found it astonishing that I can
still look young to someone when I was all dishevelled and bedrid-
den with a huge tube down my nose. Even at the height of my
cancer, my surgeon wrote in his consult on me that "this remarkably well-looking woman...has a very large colorectal tumour."
Several nurses have commented about how excellent my colour is,
so much so that they thought I did not look sick at all. Sometimes
even the other cancer patients would spontaneously exclaim, as I
walked into the chemo room, that I looked really well. Perhaps this
well-looking was part of what led those four doctors I saw in my
search for correct diagnosis to dismiss me. I suppose if you are
going to be sick, you may as well look younger!

Steve C < 10/1/2010 5:36 PM >

Happy Birthday, Robin!!

I am so happy to see that things are going well for you, even though there have been some pretty big bumps along the way. Several years ago, my brother was diagnosed with colon cancer, but his surgery was not so successful as yours. It had spread too far because he had been reluctant to go to the doctor and do what needed to be done. Since the cancer had spread so far, it was inoperable, and he had no choice but to just make the best of things. It finally took his life two years later.

You, on the other hand, have done all (and more) of the right things, and things look very promising for you. I am so happy and encouraged for you. Reading all of your emails, as you have gone through this ordeal, has been a re-living of my brother's experience for me, so it has been hard to know what to say or do.

I am so glad that your operation was successful and that you are in such great physical and mental shape. You are a poster girl for the power of positive thinking and healthy living!!

I hope you have a great rest of the day for your birthday and look forward to hearing about the rest of your recovery.

Lesley H < 10/4/2010 2:53 PM >

Happy belated birthday to you! May it bring health and healing to you and more of that tremendous courage that you have shown, as well as all of the delights of being alive. Your process sounds like it is forging such a deep appreciation of life within you. Your story helps us all reflect on what life is, and to worship it in all of its terrible beauty. Thank you for sharing your hard-won insights with me.

I send you a big hug with a squeeze and all the colours of an Eastern October forest, brilliant in its graceful transformation. Enjoy the music!!!

I have made it through the nightmare of surgery and emergency hospitalization. But another confrontation lies ahead. Doctors One through Four have responded to my College complaint. Their letters arrived while I was in hospital. It is time to open them.

14

WHEN A PATIENT COMPLAINS TO THE COLLEGE OF Physicians and Surgeons, the respondent doctor is required to counter by letter. The doctor's response is shared with the patient, who can send a final response. The doctor is also allowed one final letter in response. After these two passes, the matter can move on to investigation by one of CPSNS's two investigation committees.

When the first letters of response arrived while I was in hospital, I had wisely put them aside, knowing that I would not have the strength to address them until I had recovered from surgery. I asked the College for an extension beyond the 10 days normally afforded for response.

One week before chemotherapy is to start, I open and read their letters of defence.

Dr. One had little to say. She had been unaware of our provincial standards for *C. Difficile* testing. She had recently come from another province, and she had never had problems with such testing before. She did not order a scope or talk to me about the possibility of cancer because she considered such an outcome "statistically unlikely" in a 46-year-old. In her view, it was my responsibility to chase down my own test results. Even though negative or positive results would require followup, she did not book a return appointment for me because she saw this as the responsibility of Doctor Two. She indicated that she was now aware of our provincial screening standards for colorectal cancer and would use them in the future.

Dr. Two admitted that she had omitted my immediate family history of colorectal cancer from her referral letter. She also acknowledged that she left out her own exam and test results. However, she did not address her other serious omissions, such as leaving out any mention of the "bloody tissue" she had documented in her EMR notes. She stated that she was aware of appropriate C. *Difficile* testing standards, but had forgotten them at the time. She apologised for my frustration at being sent for the wrong test a second time. When her practice closed, she had sent a generic letter to all local specialists including Dr. Four: in her view, this was adequate for continuity of care. She did not warn me about the potential seriousness of my symptoms, even though she was leaving me without a doctor, because she "was not in the habit" of such discussions without more testing.

Dr. Three described his reason for taking no action in response to my visit with him. He had read Dr. Two's letter and decided that an appropriate referral had already been made. Bloodwork ruled out celiac disease as the cause of my bleeding; thus, he judged me to be "systemically well" at the time. Because his electronic records indicated that he had "completed" the call to Dr. Four when such a call was never made, he had asked the computer company who maintained his EMR to examine it for flaws. As for his secretary blowing off my call for help, she recorded all clinically relevant calls, and they could find no evidence of my July call saying I was worse.

I find Dr. Four's response shockingly arrogant. Although she condemned all the family doctors for not correctly informing her of my status, she said it would have made no difference if they had. Even if she had known of my immediate family history or my other details, her interpretation of screening guidelines would still make me a "low-risk case." She wrote: "the usual wait time for non-urgent cases to be seen is 12 to 18 months." Without qualm, she stated that all her surgical triage was done by her receptionist, and that it was "not her practice" to notify family doctors of her excessive wait times. She said that they all should have been aware already, due to experience of inordinate waits with other patients. She was never informed of my phone calls, but would not have returned them anyway—she is "far too busy for that." As for the bleeding and pain I came to her with, she minimized such symptoms as "very common." She doubted that I had been bleeding as much as I claimed, as I was "not pale" when she saw me. She acknowledged misreading the year of my bloodwork, but she said this was of no consequence, as my terrible outcome would have been the same. She scoffed at my statement that other local surgeons saw symptomatic patients promptly. Dr. Four did not even spell my name correctly throughout her response.

With my scar still throbbing, with the threat of another obstruction looming, and with the challenge of debilitating chemotherapy ahead of me, I take on the task of responding to each doctor. Sick and damaged as I am, I am determined. Once again, I gather relevant documents, check research and citations, and pour over medical practice guidelines.

For Dr. One, I could only restate Dr. McIntyre's words: Dr. One needed to be reminded that anyone, at any age, can get cancer. Although she considered cancer "statistically unlikely," I argued that a physician's intervention should be based on the patient in front of him or her, not on statistics. Dr. One's response acknowledged that she was unaware of the CRC cancer detection guidelines at the time she saw me, unaware of provincial testing standards for *C. Difficile*, and unaware of the wait times for a scope in our region. Although I appreciated her acknowledgement of these gaps in her knowledge, I found it deeply disturbing that a licensed family physician would not know these things. Knowing it would be considered a "he said/she said" issue, I stated again that I had told Dr. One about my immediate family history of cancer. I emphasized that she ought to have booked a scope or at least a return appointment, given my documented symptom of blood mixed with stool, regardless of her differential diagnosis.

For Dr. Two, I acknowledged her frank admission of omitting my family history and her own exam results from her referral to the specialist. However, I also underscored that there were many other significant details she omitted: my previous bowel history, the severity and duration of my bleeding, and the fact that I was passing tissue as well as blood. Dr. McIntyre had told me that losing skin and flesh from the bowel can be a sign of a villous adenoma, a precancerous state. The patches of bloody skin I had told her about were actually the result of me shedding the mucosa, the innermost lining of the rectum. If Dr. Two had intervened promptly, perhaps I could have avoided cancer altogether. Dr. Two's failure to recognize the seriousness of my symptoms was compounded by her failure to communicate them to the specialist. Although Dr. Two had done bloodwork, some of which had been concerning, Dr. Two did not send along any of these results to Dr. Four. Moreover, she did not share with me the possible dangerousness of my symptoms, leaving me profoundly disempowered. Every symptomatic patient, I wrote, deserves to be told what their symptoms may signify, even if those explanations are potentially frightening. This kind of communication becomes even more crucial when the physician is abandoning the patient by closing her practice.

For Dr. Three, I produced my phone records from July, clearly showing my calls to his office, and those made immediately afterwards to Dr. Four. If his receptionist was trained to record clinically relevant calls, why had she failed in my case? I pointed out that Dr. One's and Two's electronic records described months of bleeding, which in his own note he described as "days" of bleeding. How could a family physician deem a patient with a 7-month history of passing blood and tissue rectally to be "systemically well?" Surely, when a patient presents with a potential cancer symptom, benign bloodwork that rules out alternative explanations is a reason for *alarm*, not complacency. None of my escalating symptoms or positive test results had been communicated to the specialist, despite his promises and despite my own calls. I emphasized that Dr. Three's errors were not mere technical or clerical mistakes—he had shown an avoidant approach to medicine in my case.

For Dr. Four, I underscored my horror at her abdicating decision-making regarding surgical triage to her clerical staff. I disputed her dismissive claim that I had been a "low risk" patient and attached scientific papers clarifying an immediate family history as a risk criterion. Dr. Four and her receptionist were wrong to apply screening guidelines intended for average-risk *asymptomatic* patients to those with active symptoms and an immediate family history. I attached an affidavit from my husband, who was witness to Dr. Four's avowal that the wait list in Halifax was even longer than hers. I also attached two affidavits from young people in their 20s, both of whom had been scoped within weeks of their symptom onset by other Valley specialists during the months I had waited. So Dr. Four believed I could not have been bleeding? I produced the photograph of my bulging and bleeding tumour. My tumour was the approximate mass of a grapefruit, and yet she missed it on two rectal exams. Yet Dr. McIntyre had described it as "easily palpable," both before and after the radiation had shrunk it. Perhaps, I suggested, she needed to learn his exam technique.

All four responded again. Dr. One reported that she had improved her practice by now asking about family history when seeing symptomatic patients. Dr. Two minimized the significance of her omissions: she did not see why they had delayed my specialist consult. Dr. Three, stung by Dr. Four's accusations, provided evidence from his practice that the longest recorded wait on record for Dr. Four had been eight months—he had no way to anticipate that the wait would be 18 months. He described changes he had made to his practice: from henceforth, he would read his patients' files, follow up with specialists, and have his secretary notify him if patients call in distress. Dr. Four grudgingly agreed that she would henceforth comply with CPSNS guidelines requiring specialists to communicate their wait times to family doctors. She had assumed that the wait times throughout the province were as long as her own because she had heard her colleagues complain about their wait times. It seems that Dr. Four could not resist a final dig: she was sure she had mentioned cancer when discussing possible diagnoses, but perhaps she had used language that was too sophisticated for me, misled by my seeming "intelligence."

As I work over the complaint documents, a metaphor arises in my mind that captures my perception of how their individual and collective errors brought about my catastrophe. Dr. Two had been a bad thrower. Dr. Four had been a bad catcher. Dr. Three had been the monkey-in-the-middle who slept through their game. Dr. One had never even entered the ball park. And me? I had been waiting in the dugout, oblivious. I had been forsaken, and I had not known it.

Many nights I find myself ruminating in inchoate anger towards these doctors. I lapse into unproductive fantasies of all four of them getting cross-examined by lawyers, of them being compelled to tell their story to a class of aghast medical students, of them being struck with shame that their casual negligence has resulted in the needless suffering and possible death of a patient and colleague. This brooding is particularly strong when I lie awake in the middle of the night. I work hard to push the bitterness from my thoughts, as I need to focus on healing; but sometimes, particularly when reminded by my physical pain, I find it challenging to do so.

I am particularly heartbroken by the personal betrayal of Doctors Two and Three. I had been their colleague as well as their patient. I had thought that they considered me a person: someone with a face, a name, a family. I had assumed that somehow our collegial relationship meant something to them, and it would mean that I would get adequate care. But the College investigation process revealed to me that I was mistaken. It seemed that neither doctor saw me that way. The idea that our relationship would make a difference was an idea only in my mind—it was never in theirs. To them, I had always been just another member of the audience.

Reviewing the apparent negligence of all four doctors is painful and provoking, but it is also enlivening. Far from exhausting me, taking on the challenge of responding to this complaint has bestirred my will to live. *I need to see this complaint through,* I think, *even if it is the last thing I ever do.*

I am scheduled to see Dr. McIntyre for a post-operative appointment. My pathology results are in. Maybe those thoughts are darkly prophetic.

15

DISCOURAGING NEWS

posted by Robin McGee, Tuesday, October 12, 2010, 7:00 PM

Hello RCO:

Today we saw my surgeon. Pathology had come back, and the results were worse than previously thought. Four of nine lymph nodes tested positive, which makes my stage IIIC—the worst you can be before the incurable stage IV. There is a dividing line between invasion of three lymph nodes and invasion of four. Four puts me in a higher stage with a significantly worse prognosis. He still estimates my chances of being alive in five years to be slightly higher than 50% once I go through chemotherapy. The cancer was "moderately differentiated," which is sort of medium as far as aggressiveness is concerned.

We are discouraged. I knew that my lymph was involved, just not so much. We had hopes after the surgery that the lymph was okay, as he said they looked okay, but of course the lab is the final authority.

I tell myself that I have heard the worst news I will hear for awhile, and it is not that far off from what I had known already.

In another touching story of a good doctor...the surgeon recommended I get my urine checked to see if I had a UTI or simply pain from surgery. We stopped by my new doctor's office, but it was closed. I went to wait in the ER of the Eastern Kings Memorial Community Health Centre, while Andrew appealed to the kindness of the Wellwoods, the doctors in the office next door to Dr. Good. Dr. Heather Wellwood kindly agreed to see me and tested me on the spot. Sure enough, I had an infection, and she wrote me a script right then. She and I have worked together on cases for years. She even looked tearful when she learned of my advanced cancer. It is so amazing to me to meet with caring physicians who go above and beyond the call of duty, after years of unspeakable indifference from others.

On a brighter note, the seaside cabin was lovely. I hope everyone had lots of turkey, as I did.

Karen D < 10/12/2010 8:48 PM >

Dear Robin,

You are dealing with some pretty disappointing news today. I'm sorry there is even more on your "platter." (I am convinced most of the women I know have not managed a full plate for years—we've all moved on to full platters).

I was concerned to "read" the tone in this last update and I know that you have gotten some of the worst news from the surgeon today since the initial diagnosis was made.

However, here is something I know to be true—what you now know you are up against is no more than what your body was already fighting, but now it has a shape and a name. Stay the course, Robin. Continue to reach out for help when you need it. Keep your strength and energy intact for you and the upcoming chemo. Lean on others. Not by accident you have a very strong network to support you (one you built daily with every gesture and kindness, as you went about your life for the last many years).

Davina M < 10/12/2010 8:29 PM >

I know I haven't been involved too much with you, Robin, but you are in my prayers. It seems you take three steps forward and ten back. What inspires me is your courage and your matter-of-factness. All I can say is keep fighting. You are inspiring a lot of us.

Susan B < 10/13/2010 6:54 AM >

I'm just reading your email this morning bright and early here at school, where it seems like I pretty much live these days. It will be nice once our behavior plan meetings have been completed. They seem endless here at times.

I am so sad to read about your discouraging news this morning. I guess that sometimes prayers, best wishes, and love from family and friends must seem like no match for destiny. I think of you and your family all of the time and admire the strength and resilience that you have all shown and, I am sure, will continue to put forth. I know that my prayers will continue and I will not lose the faith that you will continue to be strong in body and in spirit.

I too pray for strength for your family, your beloved husband and son in particular, as they try to make sense of this and continue to support you on this journey.

I wish that there was something that I could do, say, or pray for that would make you better. I would love to come and see you sometime if that would be okay. I know that I do not know you like others do, but I do still care. I would only come for a short time and only if you are feeling up to it.

I must get back to the day at hand. Take care, Robin, and thank you for taking so many of us on this journey of hope. It has not ended, and though the news is discouraging, I know that your fans will not waver. You can be sure of that!

Debbie M < 10/13/2010 9:54 AM >

That is very disturbing news. I'm really sorry to hear it, as are Gerry and Chris. (Nick doesn't know yet). How are you doing? I guess it means that the fight ahead is going to be tougher than we thought—what is the WW2 analogy we should use?

Poor Andrew and Austin, Mom and Dad, Jan, Gail—well really, all our family—everyone will be upset today. But we'll just have to buck up and be supportive! Did he give you a schedule for beginning chemo?

Thea B < 10/13/2010 8:19 AM >

My Sweet Robin,

Just another speed bump, which you will fly over with grace and determination.

Suzy and John < 10/13/2010 10:23 AM >

Dearest Robin,

It is certainly like being on an emotional rollercoaster. We were all heartened after surgery—and maybe it's just good old denial, the most powerful of coping strategies, but I can't but think that you are going to survive and flourish. We all love you and are hoping for the best outcome after chemotherapy. Love to Andrew and Austin.

Sonya M < 10/13/2010 12:07 PM >

Chin up, girl!! I can only imagine how it must be to hear such news, but this is the time to dig real deep and draw on all that support that you have around you. And maybe funny movies and/or the pageantry and slime of *The Tudors*!

Marla D < 10/12/2010 9:27 PM >

I am so sorry to hear the crappy news from the surgeon. That news, however, doesn't change the fact that you are an atypical woman, unlike any other. Therefore, the stats are nothing more than numbers—you are a survivor and you will beat those damn stats!!!!

Glad to hear you are having some good experiences with more of the medical professionals. Maybe it will make up for some of the less-than-stellar physicians you have seen.

Keep those emails coming. I think of you often (in fact, I was in a meeting today and insisted that we include the frequency of the student's observed behaviour because "Robin taught me to do it that way.")

Paula M < 10/12/2010 9:36 PM >

I am sorry for this setback. I, too, am discouraged for you. You have such a strong and beautiful spirit. Don't let this bump in the road weaken that. Don't give up hope.

If the hope gets heavy, let us help you carry it.

Grace M < 10/13/2010 2:07 PM >

Dear Robin,

My heart is breaking. I feel so sad. May all our thoughts of support help you at this challenging time.

My husband Steve went through this stage with his cancer. Everything looked great during Steve's surgery, but pathology results showed cancer in the lymph system as well as in the tissue out of the prostate. This was the lowest time of his "cancer walk" so far.

At the next Relay For Life after his cancer surgery, Steve looked healthy. He ran the survivor lap in Middleton because he wanted people to see that a cancer survivor can return to the preferred activities with the same joy and vitality that one had before the diagnosis.

I hope that you heal quickly and fully so that you can have a happy, active, and fulfilling life. There may be cancer on the inside, but you can do all the things that you love to do each day.

Steve knows that he will not live forever—there is cancer in his body. He does try to do lots everyday. Since 1992, Steve has been checking off the items on his "bucket list." It is amazing the things that he has done.

If you ever want to talk with Steve, just let us know. He has walked the similar walk from the positive optimism of good observations during surgery to the devastating news when the bad pathology report came back.

Do take care! My thoughts are with you!!

Stefani H < 10/14/2010 9:53 AM >

You have shared so much of this experience with us all, Robin, and your update on Tuesday was so characteristic of your balanced approach of integrating difficult information and processing things as you move along. With knowledge comes choice of actions and reactions. Hang in there and remember the outliers! There is no reason to not assume/aim for outlier status. I am looking forward to some chat and wine with you and the girls, if that fits with your agenda.

Linda G < 10/18/2010 9:31 AM >

Robin, I lift your name up in prayer. He has outstretched arms and I hope you feel His gentle, loving embrace today...He is the source of all miracles and all love...He loves challenges and He loves showing us how much He cares by taking on those challenges. Bad circumstances make what He does with it all the more amazing...His strength and courage are so reflected in how you are handling all of this...you reflect His glory in all you are doing... He will reward this obedience. You're healed and you are saved in the most important ways.

As we both know, statistics are pretty good for the group average but never can be relied on for the individual cases. We can't put too much importance on scientific knowledge...we both know how flawed that can be...and more importantly, He has a very special plan for you. I think of the strength and grace His Spirit has given to you and the example you are being for so many people...and the people in their lives that they share your story with...He is using all of this for His good. And in all of it, He's right there for every step of the way. His love for you is evident in all of this. The times I've faced the ugly and brutal, I also remembered that He doesn't give us more than we can handle. Knowing He was trusting me to find the way through it, and to lean more into Him to find that path, made me proud that He trusted me enough to allow the challenges to come my way...It's the faith He has for our hearts...finding love in the darkest of places...He's blessed you with a loving family, a great husband and amazing son...the blessings will continue. And so will my prayers.

....

Although I am shaken by his news, I remain inexpressibly thankful to Dr. McIntyre. I have the report from the surgery, written by the resident who had assisted him during the procedure. Throughout the document, the resident has used the word "carefully" to describe the exactitude and delicacy of Dr. McIntyre's actions during the operation.

I weep with gratitude as I read it, moved to think that any doctor would treat me *carefully*.

16

As I digest the seriousness of my pathology, I also seek information. The only treatment I have left to undergo is chemotherapy. I have to find the most aggressive protocol I can.

I call the Colorectal Cancer Association of Canada. Their Director of Education and Clinical Information explains that the standard of care in most places is a combination chemotherapy called FOLFOX. She sends me the Ontario practice standards, which clearly indicate that this treatment regimen is recommended for those with a high risk of recurrence.

I spend hours researching. Cancer cells need DNA and RNA to grow. Without them, the cell cannot divide. Many chemotherapy agents act to interfere with cell division. In 1957, a team of researchers led by Charles Heidelberger developed Fluorouracil, also known as 5FU. Fluorouracil is typically accompanied by the folate vitamin Folinic Acid, also called Leucovorin. This vitamin increases the power of 5FU. Together, 5FU and Leucovorin metabolize or break down into chemical agents that incorporate themselves into the cancer cell, where they inhibit the creation of DNA and RNA. Research supported the efficacy of this combination treatment—the results of several clinical trials in the sixties and seventies showed that 5FU/LV reduced mortality in stage III colon cancer patients by 33 percent. Hence, 5FU/LV has been the mainstay of chemotherapy for colorectal cancer for the past 50 years. In one of the heartbreaking footnotes in the history of cancer, Dr.

Heidelberger was himself to die of the metastatic version of the disease from which he saved millions.

In 1976, Japanese researcher Yoshinori Kidani discovered Oxaliplatin, a derivative of platinum. It was found to have a cyto-toxic effect on DNA synthesis in cancer cells. Research over the 80s and 90s confirmed its status as an effective agent against colorectal tumours. Oxaliplatin appeared to have both unique and potentiating power, so that it enabled 5FU/LV to do a better job as well as packing its own punch.

The FOLFOX chemotherapy regimen includes a combination of three agents: Folinic Acid (FOL), Fluorouracil (F), and Oxaliplatin (OX). Initial studies showed that FOLFOX improved the survival times of those with metastatic colorectal cancer undergoing this combination. Consequently, researchers wanted to know if it would improve the outcomes survival of those at lesser stages of cancer—stages II and III.

Cancer researchers are interested in many things when they study a drug. The outcome variable they are most often interested in is called "overall survival." This is unambiguous: is the patient alive or not at a certain time interval after treatment? Studies typically examine overall survival at three or five years post-treatment. But another index is "disease-free survival." Has the patient lived without relapse or recurrence? After a particular treatment, what percentage of those treated are likely to be free of disease after three years? After five years? Research on survival has suggested that if a cancer patient can make it to five years, he or she can often make it to ten years. If a patient can make it to ten years without a recurrence of cancer, he or she is considered cured.

Unlike colon cancer, rectal cancer is difficult to study. The treatment path through colon cancer is straightforward—surgery is followed by chemotherapy. However, the treatment of rectal cancer is complicated by the possible presence of other treatments, such as radiation. Our colons swim around in our bodies. Because it is constantly in motion, it is difficult to pinpoint a colon tumour with a radiation beam. In contrast, rectal cancers are fixed. They can be radiated, and so they often are in order to shrink them prior to surgery. Consequently, rectal cancer patients can have many treatments—radiation prior to or after surgery, with or without additional drugs to potentiate the radiation. All that is "noise" to researchers. Colon cancer was the focus of the first FOLFOX studies because it was cleaner and easier to study.

In 2004, a host of researchers led by Thierry Andre published a landmark study in *The New England Journal of Medicine*. They took 2246 colon cancer patients, all of whom had their stage II or stage III cancers completely removed surgically. The patients were randomly assigned to one of two possible treatments: 5FU plus Leucovorin, which was the conventional treatment, or to the FOLFOX treatment. Patients were assessed before randomization, every two weeks during treatment and then every six months for five years. They followed the patients with the ambition to discern which group had better disease-free survival. The study was conducted across 146 major international cancer treatment centres— hence the name of the study: the Multicenter International Study of Oxaliplatin/5FU-LV in the Adjuvant Treatment of Colon Cancer, also known as the "MOSAIC" study. In addition to studying survival, they also examined the relative toxicity of the protocols in terms of both short- and long-term side effects.

The results were unequivocal. Those patients receiving Oxaliplatin in addition to 5FU/LV alone had better outcomes on virtually every index. Across all stages, disease-free survival was improved, but this difference was particularly marked for patients with stage III disease: 72.2% of those given Oxaliplatin lived, compared to 65.3% who did not get it. Taken together with information on rates of relapse and recurrence, the data suggested a 23 percent reduction in the risk of relapse.

These results changed the cancer world. FOLFOX became the mainstay of colon cancer treatment for stage III colon cancer patients everywhere: the United States, Western Europe, New Zealand, and Australia. Studies on the cost-benefits of FOLFOX treatment, factoring all costs as well as quality and quantity of life in survivors, clearly indicated that despite its toxicity, FOLFOX was worth it. The years of life saved were worth the cost difference with 5FU/LV.

My research reveals that most major centres endorse FOLFOX as a treatment for rectal cancer as well. Two common-sense factors influenced that judgment: the fact that the two cancers have the same histology, and the fact that they metastasize to the same places. Ontario's guidelines made this argument clearly.

To really study a drug, researchers must randomly assign patients to a new treatment and the old treatment. The Ontario guidelines made the point that FOLFOX for rectal cancer was so universally used, no one would ever do that study. The major clinical trials currently underway did not even have an arm for 5FU/LV alone because no one was willing to randomly assign patients to a condition considered obviously inferior. Despite the international consensus, I occasionally come across sentences in the papers I read that remind me that there is no direct evidence for FOLFOX for rectal cancer.

I call the Cancer Centre. I leave a message with my nurse Lynn: please ask Dr. Dorreen to consider FOLFOX in my case. I am obviously at high risk, and I am young and strong enough to endure it. She replies that the clinical record shows that Dr. Dorreen has no plans to change my regimen from ordinary 5FU. I groan inwardly. *Why does everything have to be a fight?*

I send Dr. Dorreen a fax declaring my willingness to take on the more toxic FOLFOX regimen:

20 October 2010

Dear Dr. Dorreen:

I am sending this fax to you in advance of our consultation appointment tomorrow.

This is the Ontario practice guideline to which I was directed by the Colorectal Cancer Association of Canada regarding the recommendation for FOLFOX for my stage IIIC rectal cancer.

Page 3 makes the recommendation that patients with resected rectal cancer at similarly high risk of systemic recurrence should be offered the same systemic adjuvant therapy as their counterparts with resected colon cancer.

The rationale for this statement is found in the Discussion section of their systematic review, which I have appended as the last page of this fax.

I am very anxious to discuss these matters with you, in view of the fact that preoperative chemoradiation did not downstage my stage IIIC colorectal cancer.

RECOVERY DU JOUR
posted by Robin McGee, Tuesday, October 19, 2010, 4:45 PM

Hello RCO:

I continue to mend. The VON nurse says my incision is good enough for them to discontinue their visits. My painkiller use has drastically dropped off—I often forget all about them. Today Andrew and I walked vigorously for about an hour outside. It is astonishing how much a person can heal from a massive surgery in only five weeks.

Special thanks to many! To Marylin C, who helped me Feng Shu my closet, and to Birdie B, Caroline W, Wendy-Lee H, and Pam S for gardening extraordinaire, and to Alison L, who provided the biscuits that fueled us!

I am somewhat apprehensive today. The Colorectal Cancer Association of Canada people have strongly advised me to pursue a FOLFOX chemo regimen. This means 5FU, which I have taken before, with Oxaliplatin, another agent. This regimen has proven hugely successful for colon cancer. Ontario practice guidelines strongly recommend it for rectal cancer. My NS oncologist has said he does not follow those guidelines; he will only give me 5FU alone. We will have to thrash it out when I see him on Thursday. I dread having to challenge him, but I want THE MOST aggressive regimen he could possibly provide. I feel that I am young and strong enough to withstand it. I have downloaded all the Ontario guidelines and the research that backs them up. I wish this was easier.

I talked to my cancer care nurse today explaining my fears. She was sympathetic, particularly in view of the experiences I have had with my assessment doctors. She told me that she was so moved by my assessment story that she keeps it on her desk at all times, even though I gave it to her in June. My surgeon's nurse said the same thing—she said, "A story like yours stays with a person for a long, long, time." In any case, I will report back on Thursday to tell you all how it goes with him.

....

It is the night before we see Dr. Dorreen. I cannot sleep. Earlier that night, I had printed the MOSAIC study paper, as well as the Ontario treatment guidelines. I feel sick with apprehension.

As we drive in the next morning, I stare at the bleak landscape flashing past my window. Underneath my fog of misery and sleepless exhaustion, I feel a stirring, like a kindly tug upon my consciousness. It is a soft, probing feeling of benign intention, like a message telling me that everything will be all right, no matter what happens.

"He has something for you," Lynn says as she reviews me prior to our appointment with Dr. Dorreen. "Something he wants to show you."

When Dr. Dorreen comes in, he seems grave and quiet. He hands me a photocopied paper cribbed from the Internet. It was an undated selection from an *UpToDate* medical review. He had highlighted the words with a yellow highlighter: "Whether Oxaliplatin is beneficial for adjuvant treatment of rectal cancer is not yet established...Despite the lack of data, guidelines from the National Comprehensive Cancer Network (NCCN), an alliance of 21 of the world's leading cancer centers, include FOLFOX as an acceptable regimen for chemotherapy in rectal cancer...Although this a popular approach based upon results from the MOSAIC study in colon cancer, physicians should be aware that there is no evidence that FOLFOX is better than fluoropyrimidine therapy alone in the adjuvant setting for rectal cancer."

"I know about these arguments," I say. "I know that there is no direct evidence for Oxaliplatin with rectal cancer. But the colon cancer research—the MOSAIC study—shows how much more effective it is with advanced disease like mine. I would really like to do FOLFOX. Dr. Dorreen, I am strong enough for it. I am only in my 40s. I still have a kid at home."

I become tearful. "You've seen my pathology. Four out of nine lymph nodes were positive. I am stage IIIC, and that was *after* chemoradiation. My tumour was not downstaged by it—you know how bad a prognosis that is."

Dr. Dorreen looks miserable. "I have known people where *every* lymph node was positive," he replies, "and they are still walking around."

A hard knot of grief arises in my throat. It is hard to get my words past it.

"Please let me do FOLFOX," I beseech him. "I know it's tough. I know it requires a portacath. But I will endure anything for a better chance at survival. *Anything.*"

Dr. Dorreen hangs his head and stares down at the surface of his desk. "There is no direct evidence for the use of FOLFOX in rectal cancer," he answers bleakly. "And we practice evidence-based medicine here."

"But you know there will *never* be direct evidence!" I rail. "Everyone everywhere—all the major centres—have moved on to using FOLFOX for people at my stage. Even the clinical trials over the past five years, they don't..." I am choking now, crying openly. "...They won't even study 5FU alone anymore, no one will randomly assign people to that condition...they consider that unethical...no one will ever do that study..."

I hold out the Ontario guidelines and the research papers I collected, the papers shaking in my hand. "You *know* this—you *know* what the MOSAIC study said. FOLFOX offers a better survival chance over 5FU. Especially for someone at my stage," I sob. "I am begging you—*begging you*—to give me any chance at that."

"I know what the MOSAIC study said," Dr. Dorreen answers patiently, hollowly. "I was there when they first presented it. And I know about the Ontario guidelines. I am leaving for Ontario for a conference this afternoon."

"Then you *know* that it is considered best practice everywhere! You know what Ontario says: that colon cancer and rectal cancer are the same disease—they have the same histology, they metastasize to the same places..."

Dr. Dorreen's gentle face is suffused with pity. "I am aware of all those arguments," he answers.

"You *know* my terrible assessment story, Dr. Dorreen," I plead. "You *know* how much time I have lost against this tumour due to all that medical mismanagement. Please give me a chance to make up for that. I am young, I can take it—I want the most aggressive response you can give me."

Dr. Dorreen raises his head slowly and looks up at me. His eyes are desolate.

"Even if I wanted to give this to you," he says, very carefully, "I could not."

I stare at him, uncomprehending.

"FOLFOX is not authorized for use with rectal cancer in Nova Scotia. It is only authorized for use with colon cancer."

I stare back at him, stunned.

Andrew and I exchange glances. There is a beat of silence in the room.

"Oh my God," I breathe. "I did not know that."

He waits for us to process his statement.

"I thought..." I stumble, "I thought all along that it was up to you—I had no idea. Not approved for rectal cancer? But how can this be in the face of all the evidence?"

"That evidence is considered indirect. The MOSAIC study only involved colon cancer patients. We don't have direct studies for rectal cancer patients. So FOLFOX is not authorized in this province for patients like you."

I am reeling. "But why...? If other provinces have done it?"

Andrew and I stare at each other and then look back at Dr. Dorreen. *Even after decades of practice with breaking bad news to heartbroken people,* I think, *he looks genuinely moved and sorry.*

"Maybe I should move to Ontario?"

"If you did, it would take three months to enter the Ontario system," Dr. Dorreen warns emphatically. "You *cannot wait that long* for chemotherapy," he adds firmly.

"So what...what happens now?" I feel lost, bereft of my best hope.

"What I can do is forward your case to an internal committee to see if they will make an exception for you. This is the Oncology Review Committee, which decides on requests that fall outside the provincial formulary. I think you will have to accept that an exception is very unlikely. In the meantime, I think we have to proceed with a therapy for you."

"I can offer you two choices," he continues. "You can have infusions of 5FU intravenously. Or you could take an oral medication, Xeloda. It is a pill that converts into 5FU in the body. Studies with colon cancer patients show that this oral chemotherapy is as least as good as taking the infusional kind."

"Chemo in pill form?" I try to re-orient to his words. "How would that play out?"

"You would take it morning and night for two weeks, then off for one. You would do eight cycles."

And now for the question that every cancer patient asks, I think. "What would you recommend, if it were you?"

"If it were me, I would go with the Xeloda. Again, it is at least as effective as the 5FU and has far fewer side effects. We are having nice success with it."

"No going to hospital?" I say, realization dawning. "Could I travel?" *Maybe I can see my family this Christmas.*

"You will need to be followed up each cycle. Every other cycle you would come here, but the others will be done by telephone. So it saves you coming here as often, but you are actually followed up intensively. So yes, you can travel."

"If I start on this drug, and later the review committee grants me the opportunity to do FOLFOX, can I switch over?"

"There would be no problem with that."

Dr. Dorreen bends over the desk to compose the script. "I will submit your request to the Oncology Review Committee tomorrow. I think they meet in about three weeks."

"Can I write them or make any arguments on my own behalf to them?"

"No...and I would get in trouble if you did that."

"Trouble?"

"Trouble for involving the patient in an internal decision. They have to decide based on arguments submitted by the oncologists in the case."

"So what will you put forward to make the argument for me?" I ask.

He looks thoughtful. "We could use the Ontario guidelines. We could start with that. But please understand that there is very limited funding for chemotherapy, and exceptions to the formulary are very rarely made."

After he had gone, Lynn comes in.

"How are you doing?" she asks tentatively, seeing my tear-stained face. She listens sympathetically when she hears the outcome of our meeting with Dr. Dorreen.

"It is very, very hard on doctors like him," she says, "when they have to say no to patients regarding medications they know would be best, but are not funded here."

I have a flashback to a session I once had with a parent newly informed of her toddler's autism. I remember that mother sagging into my arms and sobbing, begging me to provide her little child with the early intervention programs offered in other provinces. I recalled my misery, having to tell her that Nova Scotia had no such programs. I nod to Lynn to convey my understanding.

"Don't hold out hope for the special exception committee," Lynn continues. "In all the time I have been here, I have seen only one exception granted. That was to a man whose tumour was right on the border of rectum and colon, so they could not really tell where it originated. He is the only rectal case I know of that got FOLFOX."

"So let me get this straight," Andrew says. "There is a dividing line between the rectum and the colon. A tumour with identical histology that is millimetres below that line does not get FOLFOX, but a tumour millimetres above that line does."

"That's right, as crazy as that sounds," Lynn confirms.

"And let me get this even more straight...we are talking adjuvant treatment—treatment *after* the tumour has been removed surgically. So all the relative positions are moved. Even that dividing line itself is gone, cut out with the tumour during surgery, so only colon tissue remains. But the decision regarding chemotherapy depends upon the *original position* of these *removed* body parts?"

"Yes, that's right"

"Technically," Andrew continues, "Robin no longer has a rectum—all she has is colon left. Are we not trying to prevent a recurrence in colon tissue? So if the government allows FOLFOX for colon cancer patients, why would they refuse it to people who only have colons?"

"I know it makes no sense to you," she sympathizes. "But it is how they do it here. In the meantime, we have started giving most patients Xeloda for their adjuvant chemotherapy, if they have private drug coverage. It has been going very well for most of them. If you can afford it, it seems to work as well or better than the infusions."

We leave with a script and a pill container.

The chemotherapy event has begun.

17

I AM SHOCKED TO LEARN THAT THERE IS NO NATIONAL STAN-
dard of cancer care in Canada. Each province makes its own
determination regarding what therapies to fund. Living or dying
depended on where you lived. Had I stayed in Ontario and never
come to Nova Scotia to work, I could receive the recommended
best-practice treatment without question.

I must go back to the drawing board to research the apparent
hole in Nova Scotia's oncology practice relative to the rest of the
world. I study the history of Oxaliplatin in Canada and Nova Scotia.
What I learn surprises me.

I learned that Oxaliplatin had a troubled history in Canada. The
manufacturer, Sanofi-Aventis, did not file for patent in Canada.
Consequently, it could not receive a "Notice of Compliance (NOC)"
by Health Canada. In the context of the incomplete intellectual
property protection pertaining in Canada before October 2006,
Sanofi-Aventis could not submit confidential data from an extensive research and development program without running the risk
of seeing its Oxaliplatin product Eloxatin immediately become
genericized. When that situation changed, and data protection
provisions were read into law, Sanofi-Aventis could then apply for
eight years of patent protection under the new legislation.

While the rest of the world's regulators approved Oxaliplatin
(the United States Food and Drug Administration's approved it
as early as 2002), Health Canada could make Oxaliplatin available

only through a special access program. Canadians were left with a patchwork of provincial approaches to the coverage of Oxaliplatin. Whereas some provinces provided the drug (e.g., British Columbia), others such as Quebec gave approval only on a hospital-by-hospital basis. Ontario took the rigid position that as long as the drug lacked an NOC, it could not be funded. Many patients were left to the mercy of the Special Access Program, a means-tested co-pay model sponsored by Sanofi–Aventis. The lack of a patent made the drug very difficult to get. The federal government was swamped by requests from cancer patients seeking special authorization. Oxaliplatin got a bad name amongst oncologists, who were frustrated by the mountain of paperwork required to access it in the context of its scarcity in Canada. Because it was not commercially available in Canada, Canadian research and experience with it lagged behind those of other countries.

On June 2007, Oxaliplatin received a NOC for metastatic colorectal cancer, and the various federal and provincial authorities quickly reviewed the drug. Generic versions were removed from the market, and the cost of the drug increased markedly. Ontario, British Columbia, New Brunswick, and Quebec made it available as a treatment for colon and rectal cancer right away.

It was in this complicated context that the Nova Scotia system reviewed Oxaliplatin. Prior to 2005, all chemo drugs in Nova Scotia were funded by the global budget of each District Health Authority. But as costs of chemotherapies increased, this became too burdensome for regional hospitals. Chemo drugs took triple the budget space relative to other drugs. To address this problem, Nova Scotia adopted a centralized approach to the authorization and management of cancer drugs. Nova Scotia established the "Cancer Systemic Therapy Policy Committee," or CSTPC. Comprised of 23 stakeholders from across the province, this committee voted whether to recommend formulary funding for various cancer drugs.

In the spring of 2007, Nova Scotia's CSTPC reviewed Oxaliplatin or FOLFOX for the treatment of colorectal cancer. They collectively and unanimously voted to approve it for use with metastatic (stage IV) colorectal cancer—both colon and rectal. They also voted to approve it for use with curable (high-risk stage II and stage III) colon cancer patients. But they excluded access for curable rectal cancer patients. Why?

After the publication of the MOSAIC study showing its impact on colon cancer, most western nations immediately endorsed FOLFOX to cure rectal cancer as well. But because FOLFOX was adopted everywhere as a standard, studies comparing it to the lesser treatment of 5FU became impossible. No patients were willing to be assigned to the 5FU control group, and oncology researchers were not willing to assign them because they considered that action to be unethical. All the studies ended prematurely. It became clear early on that no one would ever do a major randomized control study of FOLFOX versus 5FU for rectal cancer. That ship had sailed.

But Oxaliplatin was costly, particularly in light of the manufacturer's new monopoly. And it was true that there were no major controlled studies of its use in rectal cancer. By the absolute letter of the law, there was no proof that it helped to cure rectal cancer. To doctors and bureaucrats anxious about health care costs, the "lack of evidence" provided enough of a reason to refuse endorsement.

By the time I am diagnosed in 2010, the research supporting the efficacy of FOLFOX for colon cancer had become even stronger. The same patients from the MOSAIC study had been followed for a further three years. At five years post treatment, the FOLFOX advantage remained evident for stage III patients: 66.4% for those receiving FOLFOX were still disease-free, compared to 58.9% of those who got 5FU/LV alone. This corresponded to a 20 percent reduction in the risk of relapse and death.

I post my sorry experiences, and the responses give me the germ of an idea...

DISCOURAGEMENT
posted by Robin McGee, Thursday, October 21, 2010, 3:45 PM

Hello All:

Well, today the oncologist said that the best practice treatment I learned about is not approved for use in Nova Scotia. It is allowed in most provinces including Ontario, but not here. NS uses this treatment for colon cancer, but not rectal cancer. Other provinces consider these cancers the same.

He says he will present my case to a special committee to see if they will allow an exception. But because my pathology indicated rectal cancer, he does not hold out much hope.

In the meantime, he will start me on an oral form of chemotherapy called Xeloda. This drug turns into 5FU in the body. Therefore, I will not need to get any intravenous infusions, I can travel, I avoid the hospital, etc. I start on Monday. The regimen is two weeks on, one week off—for six months. It is said to be much, much easier on patients than 5FU infusions.

We are discouraged, of course. We wonder if I should try to seek the proper treatment through a private clinic, or by moving to Ontario. I do have family there. We don't know where to start with that. Do any of you in Ontario know an oncologist?

I plan to drink some Scotch this weekend, before chemo starts. *Sigh*

Patricia M < 10/21/2010 4:19 PM >

Hi Robin. You might try calling the Minister of Health's office to appeal. And/or call your member of the provincial assembly, your MLA, and ask them to advocate for you with the Minster of Health.

I do not know any oncologists here in Ontario. I have been retired too long. You would need a referral from the NS oncologist and I think you would find there would be a long wait list.

Kym H < 10/20/2010 4:37 PM >

Oh Robin, I am so sorry that the oncologist was not in agreement with your research. I know how much this means to you and I can't imagine how upset you must have been leaving that office today. I will keep my fingers crossed that the committee will make the second exception for you. I can understand the thinking about moving to Ontario, but as you said yesterday, it may put your treatment on hold and can you do that? Perhaps your doctor friend in Ontario can find you someone and get you in right away. In the meantime, you will be starting the 5FU (does the FU stand for F--- Y---?). Having a wee nip (or giant slosh) of Scotch seems like the right way to prepare for Monday. Will you have company on Sunday? I am making a delicious squash soup and thought I would bring some up to you (it might have a wee dram of something in it. :) (Just kidding...but it does have maple syrup).

True to the scientist within me, I set to work to study the drug I had been given: Capecitabine, brand-named Xeloda.

Xeloda's star rose in the oncology heavens in 2005, after an important paper was published in *The New England Journal of Medicine*. Xeloda is a "pro-drug"; that is, in essence, it is enzymatically converted to 5FU in the tumour. Due to its action, it differentially attacks cancer cells compared to normal cells, which makes the overall regimen less prone to side effects. In the multicenter Xeloda in Adjuvant Colon Cancer Therapy or "X-ACT" study led by Chris Twelves, 1087 stage III colon cancer patients were randomly assigned to receive either oral Capecitabine or 5FU/LV. Although the gross disease-free survival after three years did not differ, more refined analyses revealed a slight superiority of Xeloda over 5FU/LV on most efficacy factors. Moreover, the study convincingly demonstrated far less toxicity with Xeloda. Since that time, Xeloda has increased in popularity among patients and oncologists, given its ease of use. No infusions, no portacath, no hospital visits, and no costs associated with those procedures. Private drug companies cover it, and Roche, the manufacturer, provides co-pay options for those who do not have full coverage.

I have strong and mixed feelings about Xeloda. On one hand, each time I take it—swallowing it by the handful when the buzzer on my phone indicates—I sigh in gratitude that it is so easy. When

I rise from the table or the couch to take it and look out the window at the winter winds racing around the house, I feel fully how much easier it is than getting into the car and driving to the hospital. I bless it for how easy it seems physically. No nausea, no GI problems. On the internet, I watch videos of how it takes action—the images show small globes descending on cancerous tissue and destroying it, while the nearby healthy tissue sparkles untouched. When I think about how it will allow me to travel to see my family this Christmas, my heart swims with gratitude. My parents are in their 80s and still living in the house I grew up in. I have an overwhelming need to see them again, fearing as I do that it may be for the last time.

Xeloda lets me be free. Xeloda lets me see friends. Xeloda lets me spend my days in other cancer-fighting pursuits, such as exercise or meditation. I am so grateful for it.

But I also resent it. Whenever I brush across the research on Oxaliplatin, I feel my gorge rise with the outrage of it—that I must settle for Xeloda because FOLFOX is denied me here. And not just me, but all the other node-positive rectal cancer patients, most of whom do not even know of their deprivation. They looked to their oncologists with perfect trust, and those oncologists looked back at them while harbouring in their hearts the knowledge that a better treatment existed. I imagine those Nova Scotian oncologists, shifting restlessly in their conference seats when presenters from other provinces and countries shared their survival rates. I imagine that small "have not" feeling that would stir beneath the surface of their thoughts any time a colleague described a clinical success with FOLFOX. I imagine their frustration as they read through the guidelines for adjuvant therapy published repeatedly in other provinces as well as in national and international journals. I imagine how sickened they felt, watching the desperate and intrepid stage III rectal cancer patients move away from Nova Scotia to get FOLFOX elsewhere. I imagined how they might brood upon the hardship and expense forced upon those despairing people, as they watch the stage III colon cancer patients arrive at the hospital to get comfortably infused with Oxaliplatin.

It does not escape me that Xeloda had no studies on it specifi-cally as an adjuvant treatment of rectal cancer—the studies had all been on colon cancer patients. But the costs of Xeloda could be offloaded to private insurance companies, thus reducing costs for the province. The double standard irks me.

Each day, I undertake the preventative measures I had been told to do. Each day and night I slather my hands with udder cream. Each day I take the supplementary B6 vitamins that Dr. Dorreen has prescribed.

I do not surrender my quest for FOLFOX. I phone every private clinic in Ontario: none of them offer it. "It is publically funded here," one explains, "so there is no market for a private clinic to provide it." The clinics I reach are shocked to learn that FOLFOX for rectal cancer is not available in Nova Scotia. The experience is sickening.

Could I move to the United States? Could I afford it? Private FOLFOX would cost me well over 50 thousand US dollars—and that would be just for the drug, not for the cost of travel and accommo-dation. But what about my family? Could I disrupt them by pulling Austin out of school or Andrew from his job? Could I fly back and forth? How safe would that be if I were immune-suppressed? Who would follow me medically?

Each day on the internet brings fresh evidence that FOLFOX would have been my best hope. I read the British Columbia guide-lines, which offered Xeloda therapy to everyone *except* those at my stage, who were *always* offered FOLFOX. Some of what I read is scalding and heartbreaking to me. For example, I read one surgi-cal journal in which the author argued that resected rectal cancer patients should not be given postoperative chemotherapy at all. In his view, it was a waste of time and money. The only exception, he said, was cancer at the IIIC level like mine. And the only therapy IIIC's should get was Oxaliplatin-based, as only FOLFOX had any hope of working for disease that advanced. After reading that paper, I have to take a walk around the block and take many, many deep breaths.

It is angering. It is nauseating. It is despairing. But I have no choice.

At night, I pour over studies that compared Xeloda to other protocols. In Europe, scientists were moving ahead with developing a protocol that combined Capecitabine with Oxaliplatin—so called "CAPOX" or "XELOX" regimens. But these are not available in North America yet. For some reason, North Americans find this regimen far more toxic than Europeans do, and at 2010 conferences oncologists have declared that it is not yet time for CAPOX in North America.

Discouraged and overwhelmed, I email the Director of Education and Clinical Information at the Colorectal Cancer Association of Canada. She wisely counsels me to consider the potentially harmful stress of interprovincial travel and the relative value of acceptance.

Director of Education and Clinical Information, CCAC
< 10/21/2010 2:44 PM >

Hi Robin:

Moving to Ontario and accessing therapy would not necessarily be a walk in the park, so to speak. There is a three-month waiting period and I don't believe that would be in your best interest. I would much rather you access Xeloda than having to wait to access FOLFOX. Having said that, when will the medical oncologist get back to you regarding the expert committee request for access to FOLFOX? If the government is not willing to fund it, will they permit you to access and pay for it? Kindly advise.

Please do not feel defeated. Accessing therapy is the most important thing for you right now and regardless of the type, therapy is indeed available to you. Let's keep a good thought about the expert committee request and take it from there. Please let me know how it goes.

Robin McGee < 10/22/2010 10:48 PM >

Hi again CCAC:

I am wondering if I could be a candidate for a CAPOX protocol...
if I take the Xeloda offered here but go to Toronto or Ottawa for the
Oxaliplatin?

Of course, I am struggling with the quality of life issue here.
Perhaps taking Xeloda alone and NOT pursuing the Oxaliplatin
outside Nova Scotia would result in more peace, and hence a
better outcome. It is hard for me to judge.

I am so frustrated that Nova Scotia is happy to prescribe Xeloda to
rectal patients based on colon cancer studies, but will not authorize Oxaliplatin.

Director of Education and Clinical Information, CCAC
< 10/22/2010 12:17 PM >

Hi Robin:

If it were me, I might be inclined to pursue the Xeloda alone if
it meant being able to achieve some peace of mind and good
quality of life. I am certain that you are aware of the important role
played by positive thinking and a stress-free life.

There haven't been any validation studies performed in Canada
on CAPOX, which would make it difficult to access. Though if you
take a look at the clinical research updates that I prepare every
month, you will see that there have been a number of studies
performed elsewhere comparing FOLFOX to CAPOX, concluding
that Xeloda is comparable to 5FU in terms of efficacy. Here is the
link to the research updates: http://www.colorectal-cancer.ca/en/
treatments/clinical-trials/

Bottom line: I would try to avoid any undue adversity and stress as
much as possible. What do you think?

I surrender to the Xeloda experience. I reason that if I am in the last months or years of my life, I want to spend them with my family.

And not all our struggles with medication are painful. Some are downright humourous.

PILLS GALORE

posted by Robin McGee, Friday, October 29, 2010, 9:00 AM

Hi All:

I am on day four on the pills and still no side effects. They say few people have any the first two cycles. Still, I am grateful for the reprieve, as I have been able to get some chores done and go for walks without undue hardship.

We have had a few funny experiences with the pills. The first day I got them, I put all 210 of them carefully into a pill dispenser that the drug company provided—a big "AM" and "PM" box with each day of the week labeled on every section. Just as I was closing the last segment, the entire box sprang into the air and pills sprayed everywhere! I shrieked like a banshee, bringing Andrew into the room. We crawled around on our hands and knees, picking up each little toxic pill and putting it back in the container; under our breath, we uttered prayers of gratitude that we do not have small children or pets in the house. We carefully counted to ensure we had them all back safe and sound. Just as Andrew went to close the last section, it happened AGAIN!! The pills sprayed all over the room! I confess I shrieked again—as loud a scream as I have ever voiced confronted with the largest spider imaginable. We carefully picked them up again, but this time two were missing. We searched and scoured and crawled and flashlighted—all to no avail. I was just about to call the pharmacy when Andrew discovered the culprits—they had bounced into a nearby bookcase! Once we had them all secured again, we were able to have a good laugh over it.

Enjoy your Friday-before-Halloween!

IN PRAISE OF AUSTIN

posted by Robin McGee, Monday, November 1, 2010, 11:45 AM

Hello All:

It is the first day of my second week of Xeloda and still no apparent side effects. I think it takes a few months before those are likely to emerge.

So many of you have emailed inquiring about how Austin is doing with everything that I thought I would put in a word of praise for him.

When I was first diagnosed, I think he was bewildered. He did not know much about the science of cancer (Why would he?), so it took a while for the seriousness of it to sink in. I also think he was shell-shocked by his grandfather's death from cancer that occurred near the same time. I think the true extent of things hit him when he saw me in hospital. I think the snarkiest teenager alive would have been overwhelmed by that ward.

But he has done his best to rise to the occasion. He has worked hard at improving his independence (he gets himself ready and out in the morning each day). He requires no reminders or monitoring about homework. He seems to be keeping up with school reasonably well. When we ask him to do a chore, he leaps up and does it right away. He is unfailingly affectionate and supportive. He has undergone all the deprivations this cancer has brought to his life without complaint. For example, each year since he was 8-years-old, we have had a birthday party for him, celebrated before Halloween, in which he films his friends in a fun movie. We have done movies about vampires, zombies, and aliens, all starring him and his friends. We had to cancel that this year, with my treatments so up in the air. He brooked losing that event with equanimity, and we have tried to make up for it by letting him have friends over. Last night several came over to help us put on our haunted show. So on the whole, I think he is handling things as well as someone his age could.

Andrew and Austin have gone in together in buying a 1962 LandRover in need of restoration. They got it on ebay, and it arrives from BC this week sometime. It will be a "Dad and the Lad" project that they will do together. Austin is very excited to have these "new" wheels arriving, and it should prove a positive distraction. Now he just has to get a job and learn to drive!

For the curious, our Halloween show was a success despite the cold drizzle. Several kids shrieked with delight at our routine, and many exclaimed "That one was the best!" as they ran down the drive to their parents. The kids would enter our inner garden, which was misty from our fog machine and covered with spooky decorations. I was dressed like a creepy raven. When they rang the doorbell, I would open it slowly and step out among them, asking them if they were here for candy. They would timidly answer "yes," and then I would turn to the house and say, "Then I must summon the Dread Lord. Come, Dread Lord!" Andrew would slowly thump towards the door, silhouetted by a strobe light, and emerge in his 8-feet-tall ghoul costume! Meanwhile, Austin and his friends manned a swinging boom from his window, so that another big ghoul flung himself down at the trick-or-treaters. Hidden teens dressed in scream masks would chase them down the driveway... all in all, a fun experience for all. Too bad it is only once a year!

Suzy and John < 11/2/2010 10:50 PM >

Why am I not surprised that Austin has managed to cope so well? Because, as you know, we are Austin Fans and have always been. I think he is one of the most interesting and remarkable and lovely kids we have ever known. Of course a little credit is due to his great parents—nobody has a spirit like Robin, and I am so grateful that we have become friends over the years. So many hugs to you all and much love.

Lesley H < 11/1/2010 1:01 PM >

What a great kid! Congratulations on what sounds like a very creepy Halloween experience!

Wanda C < 11/1/2010 2:14 PM >

Hi Robin, Andrew, and Austin:

So glad to hear that your haunted house was a success...I am in awe of your imaginations!! I remember when you lived in Coldbrook and Andrew was the "pumpkin person." As the teens arrived to get treats Andrew would rise up and scare the bejesus out of them. I am not sure of the exact words but one teen girl said that he had almost made her wet her pants! Fog machines, amazing costumes, spooky music...yes, wouldn't it be great if this could happen more than just once a year. You fellows are the best!!

Austin is a very well-rounded individual and I had no doubt that he would be a supportive son in every way...of course the fact of your diagnosis and losing his grandfather all happening so close together must have been so totally overwhelming for him as for all of you.

Robin, hopefully you will continue to do well with your medication and have little or no side effects.

Always in our thoughts and prayers.

Marilyn C < 11/1/2010 12:38 PM >

You cut me up! How anyone still has the desire for these things in your condition is more than I know, but I DO know it is this very thing that will be the reason you beat this evil disease!

Debbie M < 11/1/2010 12:33 PM >

Good thing little kids aren't prone to heart attacks!

....

I am not always fully forthcoming with RCO about my sufferings. Some of the details are too gruesome, too private. Coping with the temporary ostomy is such an issue. I have an ileostomy, a stoma in the small intestine close to the stomach. That means that the stool that is excreted through it is liquid, with the consistency of a milkshake. It is comprised largely of stomach acid.

My stoma is unstable. As I regain weight after the surgery, it becomes smaller. It tilts to the side, so that the orifice is aimed at my skin. The acidic stool acid eats through the seals and glues used to hold on the appliance in place. The stomach acid escapes: burning me, digesting me. The skin surrounding the stoma is raw and excoriated. The pain is continuous. Underneath the glues, it feels as if my skin is screaming for oxygen. Some nights the seal and appliance come off completely, and I wake up covered with my own scalding excrement.

I stink. I was told when I left the hospital I could change my appliance every five days. My seals simply do not last that long, dissolved as they are by the acid. I change it every other day. The appliances are very costly, over $10 dollars each. *What do people do who do not have a drug plan that helps cover these essential supplies?* The odour seems to follow me around all day—on my clothes, my sheets, my furniture.

They told me in hospital to sit on the toilet and empty the pouch into it. I learn quickly that this is a bad idea. I learn instead to kneel in front of the toilet and spend the stool out of the end of the pouch like a man urinating. Hard calluses develop on my knees.

The pouch must be emptied every few hours, including the small hours of the morning. I must get up with it at least three times each night. I am exhausted.

I cannot post about this ugliness. Instead, I share other serious musings:

SO FAR, SO GOOD

posted by Robin McGee, Saturday, November 6, 2010, 2:30 PM

Hello All:

So far, so good on the oral chemotherapy. No side effects at all. On Tuesday, two big things will occur: I will find out if I can get the best practice treatment for my stage, disallowed currently in NS (not much hope here), and I will be officially able to eat normally. No more low fibre! My first ambition is to eat oranges.

As we approach Remembrance Day, I am reading a book by Nevil Shute entitled *Pastoral*. It was written in 1944; it is a fictional story about an RAF bomber pilot. Reading the experiences is astonishing to me in so many ways. First, I reflect that my own father lived through these very terrors (like being damaged in combat, lost at night, and running low on fuel). My Dad was a navigator on Lancasters during WW2. Second, I am stunned by how young these men and women were. Here is a sentence from the novel that made me murmur aloud, from a conversation of a female Radio Officer with a Bomber Pilot: "She was two years older than him, being twenty-one; she felt almost motherly to him." Third, I am agog at how these fighters went up in the air in terrible peril of their lives—much greater peril even than I am in now—and did so with duty, equanimity, and resolve. Cancer is very frightening, but it cannot possibly be more frightening than war. Something to ponder as we approach Remembrance Day.

So far, so good

posted by Daphne K at Saturday, November 6, 2010, 3:23 PM

"Cancer is very frightening, but it cannot possibly be more frightening than war"...I don't know Robin; I see the parallels. The invasion of enemy cells, their attack, not knowing whether they will attack further. Attacking back with chemo and radiation, the duration of the battle, the surprise attack of a blockage after surgery, etc. It is smaller scale in comparison because one person is under attack, but it affects many more people. I could go on, but I won't.

You're the brave soldier in this battle who has an army of supporters cheering you on to stay positive in your fight to beat this enemy.

Marla < 11/6/2010 6:33 PM >

Hi Robin,

I related very strongly to your message today. I am thinking of my son, Joshua (25), who is serving in Afghanistan right now. He is expected home at the end of the month (keep your fingers crossed!!). I met some of the fellows that were being deployed with them...one was 19!!! I chatted with him at some length and noted that he was probably learning disabled (did poorly in school, liked to work with his hands...) and so much like so many of the kids I teach. What a worry.

I too am agog at the strength of the human spirit...yours and theirs.

You all inspire me to do better, be better, each day. Keep up the good work!!!

I think of you often and miss our professional (and sometimes unprofessional!) conversations.

Sheila M < 11/7/2010 2:41 PM >

As I sat here, swamped by paper work in my office, I read your email and cried.

Your thoughts of others, and your ability to think outside of the present moment, are amazing to me.

I think of you more than you will ever know and look forward to coming to see you on your next project day. I look forward to that.

Although this job keeps me at school for very long hours and at times I do get discouraged—I know that I am doing it to make a difference in ways that I might not be able to in other positions. By having had you as a model for quite some time now, I am able to see the difference that making sure what is best for students happens in a school. It is quite amazing the difference your philosophy and encouragement has made within the schools for the last number of years. Without you daring to take the lead in so may ways, I would not have the courage and opportunity to say and do the things I can do in a school to support children and their families.

That being said, I will go back to my pile of papers and work through them so I can enjoy my day tomorrow!

At home, Andrew tries to cope constructively. The LandRover he is restoring with Austin is somehow a source of self-soothing. Machines can be repaired, even if bodies cannot, and the time he spends on it feels like progress of a sort. The project provides its own mysteries to distract him. It helps Andrew to have one part of his life over which he still has some control. I am relieved to see him work with his hands again, knowing how this can channel his stress.

As I am having so few side effects, a great ambivalence arises in me. Xeloda is so *easy*. Do I really want to undergo a regimen known to be so much more toxic and harsh? That is more complicated in its delivery? That needs a portacath? That would give me another slow infusion 5FU bottle?

The more I read about FOLFOX's success relative to 5FU alone, the more the answer is "yes." I tell myself that I would do anything to get better treatment. I would be willing to take on the whole world if it would grant me a better chance to live. I already have a fight on my hands with cancer itself: now, another battle looms ahead.

18

ANDREW AND I ARE AT THE ONCOLOGY APPOINTMENT, THE first after starting Xeloda. Lynn is with us, reviewing how I have done. She is pleased when the symptom review reveals no significant problems.

"Most people who react poorly to Xeloda do so in the first cycle," she tells us. "So if you are tolerating it well now, you should be able to stay on it. Most people complain of fatigue towards the end, and some have the sore hands and feet, but if you are handling it well now, that is a great sign."

"Any news from the exception committee?" I ask.

"None that I know of." Lynn grins suddenly. "But Girl, I have something to tell you. You have stirred up a hornet's nest around here! They are talking about your case—well, not your case, but this issue of FOLFOX—in the lunchroom and in the hallways. I hear that several of the oncologists have come forward to Dr. Dorreen saying that there needs to be a change to extend it to rectal cancer."

"What does Dr. Dorreen think of this? He is the head of oncology."

"I think he favours it as well," she replies. "But you know, clinicians cannot change things just by wanting to. Even if the doctors here made a recommendation to the Department of Health, it is the politicians in the government that approve the funding—this is one for the politicians."

She leaves, telling me that she will share my details with Dr. Dorreen.

When he enters, he shakes my hand. "Nice to see you, and to see that you are doing well," he says. He sits down and looks over my recent bloodwork results.

"Your blood is just where it ought to be," he reassures me. "I will prepare another script for you."

He turns in the swivel chair to face me directly. "I have not heard back from the special committee," he says straightforwardly, "but I think the chances of them approving you for FOLFOX are slim to none. The chemotherapy budget was exceeded many months ago, and the money would have to come out of other hospital services here. I am anticipating they will turn us down."

Us? I notice his word. *Does that mean he truly supports FOLFOX for rectal cancer? Or is this a figure of speech?*

"I have called all over Ontario," I tell him. "I cannot find a clinic that will give me FOLFOX, but some will do just plain Oxaliplatin. I would need an oncologist to prescribe and to follow, as they do not provide any medical followup, just the infusions. But I am apprehensive about that, because I am not sure about how that would work or if it would be safe, particularly with the travel aspect."

"There is a private clinic in Halifax that does infusions," he says thoughtfully, "but I do not think they do chemotherapy. You could call them to check."

Is he tacitly saying that he supports my search?

"I want Oxaliplatin treatment so much, as you know," I continue, "but I do not want to take unnecessary risks. The other day, I read some 2010 conference proceedings. One of the presenters was studying the XELOXA protocols—Xeloda and Oxaliplatin combined. He said that his group found that taking Xeloda and Oxaliplatin together is too toxic for North Americans now. For some reason, we differ from Europeans. That scared me. I want the most aggressive treatment possible, but I do not want to go out on a crazy limb that no one can guide me through."

He looks concerned, is about to say something, then stands up and moves to the calendar to search for our next appointment time, his back to me.

"Could I pay for FOLFOX myself?" I plead. "Just give the province the money?"

He returns to his seat, shaking his head. "No, you cannot."

"Because that would be two-tiered medicine?"

"Yes, and because it is not approved for use with your kind of cancer here. That is what would have to change. Until that changes, neither you nor anyone else can access it."

Change, I think hopelessly. *Could there ever be hope of change?*

I sigh. "I fear suffering and death as much as the next person. I know Xeloda is easy, and FOLFOX is hard. But if I could get FOLFOX, I would embrace it despite all its hardship. If it can improve my chances of surviving, I would start it tomorrow."

Dr. Dorreen cocks his head to one side and smiles at me genially. "*You* are not going to die," he says.

....

It is night. I have taken my evening Xeloda. I sit in my chair by the fireplace, my laptop before me. I have just closed the internet window on another oppressive search on the superiority of FOLFOX.

An idea is forming, slowly, tentatively.

The government must make the changes. That is the message I have heard loud and clear.

I reflect on my own clinical experience: how nauseating it had been to tell parents of autistic preschoolers that we had nothing for them. My repeated appeals to change this unjust situation had been futile. However, the policy *did* change. Early intervention became available once those same crushed parents united and collectively lobbied the provincial government. Their tireless advocacy eventually resulted in formulary funding for early intervention for preschoolers with autism. *Maybe,* I wonder, *lobbying could change things for cancer patients too.*

For government policy to change, pressure must be applied by the public. Was I not a member of the public?

But what would happen if I tried to appeal to the government for FOLFOX? Would this anger Dr. Dorreen? In my time, I had met many a physician who would react with arrogance and outrage if a patient tried to do an end run around him or her to get improved care. What if Dr. Dorreen regarded my lobbying as a criticism or rejection of his plan for me? Would that put him at risk? What if I got him in some kind of trouble, as he indicated might happen if I personally approached the internal committee?

Maybe I should shut my mouth. I am a cancer patient on chemotherapy for God's sake—I need to be resting. Xeloda is easy and tolerable. Maybe I should just be happy with that. Just let it go, Robin.

I pull the laptop closer to me and nestle it on my lap. My fingers go to the keys. A memory circles over my thoughts like an eagle. What was that saying by the abolitionist Horace Mann? *Be ashamed to die until you have won some victory for humanity.*

Maybe I will jeopardize myself if I speak out. But I know I am not the only person at risk for premature death because they cannot access this treatment. But if I am going to die because of inadequate medicine, I will not die ashamed.

I mull over the clues Lynn had given me that Dr. Dorreen and the other oncologists endorse the extension of this therapy. If I speak out, I know that I must gamble on Dr. Dorreen's character. I will have to take a risk that, if asked, he will come out in support of this treatment.

I have been a practicing clinical psychologist for 20 years: I have been observing people's personalities for my entire career. Nothing about Dr. Dorreen strikes me as imperious or vindictive. My instincts tell me that he is a humble, well-meaning, and careful man—a man of science.

I swallow my fear. I make a leap of faith, and begin typing.

The New Democratic Party (NDP) had won the provincial election in June of 2009. They have been in power for 14 months. I know my MLA Jim Morton from a shared past. He had been at the helm of local Addictions Services for many years before his election to office. We had crossed paths several times in our roles as clinicians in the public health system. I write to him and to the Minister of Health and Wellness, Maureen MacDonald.

From: Robin McGee
To: Minister Maureen MacDonald; Jim Morton, MLA
Sent: Tuesday, November 09, 2010 6:17 PM
Subject: Authorizing FOLFOX for stage III rectal cancer

> I am a resident of Kings North. I am emailing to bring to your attention a health care issue in Nova Scotia.
>
> I am a cancer patient. I have stage IIIC rectal cancer. This cancer is curable. However, I have learned that the best-practice treatment for it is not authorized in Nova Scotia.
>
> International research has demonstrated that colon cancer is best treated with a chemotherapy called FOLFOX, which contains the ingredient Oxaliplatin. Patients with stage III colon cancer treated with FOLFOX had 20% reduction in risk of death, relative to those treated with the standard therapy (5FU) (Andre et. al. 2009, see http://171.66.121.246/content/27/19/3109.full). The research is so compelling that FOLFOX has been adopted as the best practice standard for chemotherapy among stage III rectal cancer patients as well. This is true in several provinces, including Ontario and BC, as well as throughout the United States and Europe. However, in Nova Scotia, FOLFOX is authorized for colon cancer, but not rectal cancer.
>
> The Ontario Cancer Care Guidelines summarize the research and the rationale for using FOLFOX with stage III rectal cancer (see PDF attached). These oncology experts write: "Given the biologic similarity between colon and rectal cancer in terms of their histology, tissue of origin, patterns and risk of systemic recurrence, and the fact that these two diseases are treated the same when they metastasize, the adjuvant systemic therapy of rectal cancer has been led by advances in the adjuvant therapy of colon cancer... in North America, based on the extrapolation of data from the

adjuvant colon trials, Oxaliplatin-based postoperative therapy has been accepted as a standard for rectal cancer...it is reasonable and appropriate to offer patients with resected rectal cancer at high risk of systemic recurrence the same adjuvant systemic therapy as their counterparts with colon cancer" (Evidence-based Series #2-4, Section 2, page 18).

Why is Nova Scotia falling below an internationally accepted best practice standard?

I am in my 40s. If I am cured, I will return to being a productive tax-paying citizen. If I am not, my death will be prolonged and extremely expensive. I urge the government to allow FOLFOX for the treatment of stage III rectal cancers. Not only will this save Nova Scotian lives, it will result in cost savings relative to the treatment for metastatic stage IV disease.

I hit send. Then, I reach out to the RCO community:

ONCOLOGY VISIT TODAY
posted by Robin McGee, Tuesday, November 09, 2010 6:40 PM

Hello RCO:

We saw the oncologist today. They are pleased with my lack of side effects. The nurse said that if one goes through two cycles without side effects, one typically does well. She said that fatigue arises as the cycles continue, but the other serious side effects do not if they have not manifested themselves early.

There is still no news on whether I will be permitted the superior FOLFOX treatment offered in other provinces, although it looks pretty dim. My nurse told me that my appeal to the special committee has created a debate! Apparently, several of the oncologists at Dickson are distressed about the inferiority of NS treatment; they want to approach the government to do something about it. However, my oncologist told me that it is highly likely that I will be refused for budget reasons. He said that they have already "maxed out" their chemotherapy budget and thus cannot afford exceptions.

So once again it seems my crusading may pay off for other people, but it is too late for me. There is some satisfaction in that nevertheless.

To press the issue, tonight I sent an email to my MLA and Minister of Health, urging them to allow FOLFOX for stage III rectal cancer patients. Below is the text of that email. Perhaps some of you Nova Scotians might email too. The Minster of Health is Maureen MacDonald, and her email is attached. If we all email her, she might soften when the doctors approach her.

Everyone feel free to email the government! This disease can strike you or your loved ones, so we all stand to benefit if they improve treatments here.

As I hit send, I wonder what will happen next.

19

RCO HAS RESPONDED.

My smartphone is chirping constantly. Every few minutes, I get another email from an RCO member who has copied me on their email to the Minister.

The submissions are thoughtful, developed, unique. I am astonished: the content is eulogic and heartwarming.

From: Alison Lannan
To: Maureen MacDonald, Health Minister
Cc: Jim Morton
Sent: Wednesday, November 10, 2010 6:25 PM
Subject: FOLFOX treatment

Dear Ms. MacDonald,

As a resident of the Annapolis Valley, I have had my life impacted many times by Dr. Robin McGee. Firstly, she is my next-door neighbour. Secondly, she is a school psychologist in the AVRSB, providing invaluable assistance to students, parents, and teachers. She is a leading authority in the area of attention deficit hyperactivity disorder; she has made a huge difference in the lives of many children. As a teacher, I have benefitted greatly from Dr. McGee's expertise in many areas of children and the conditions that affect their learning.

At this time, Dr. McGee is unable to work in the AVRSB as she is fighting the fight of her life versus rectal cancer. She is a highly educated person, who knows how to research and access information. Never before have these skills been so needed by her. She has researched her disease and also researched the most effective treatment recommended for it. She has, to her horror (and mine), discovered that Nova Scotia is one of the few places in the educated, Western world that does not approve the most effective treatment for her type of cancer: FOLFOX for those with stage III rectal cancer. It seems archaic to me that there exists a treatment that is proven to significantly improve a patient's chances of survival, yet is not approved in our province—a province which has opted for a lesser, significantly less effective, and cheaper treatment. This is an embarrassment and a travesty. To put money ahead of health is appalling.

The long-term cost to society of not providing FOLFOX to Dr. McGee is much greater than the cost of FOLFOX. The AVRSB needs her back desperately; we are in great need of trained school psychologists of her calibre. We, her friends, need her to be healthy, but most importantly, her 15-year-old son and her husband need her to be healthy.

I am asking you to reconsider this decision of turning Dr. McGee down for FOLFOX. I am asking the province of Nova Scotia to do what is right and pay for the most effective treatment, the treatment Dr. McGee would receive if she lived elsewhere in the country or in the Western world. Don't relegate NS to the status of poor cousin. We are better than that.

Thank you for your time,

Alison Lannan

Dear Ms. MacDonald,

I am writing as a concerned Nova Scotian. Up until recently, I have been a supporter of our health system and believed wholeheartedly that Nova Scotians were privy to some of the best medical treatments and services in our country. That was until I learned of the horrible trials and tribulations that my previous supervisor and mentor, Dr. Robin McGee, has endured over the past few years. Dr. Robin McGee is one of the kindest, happiest, and optimistic people I have ever met. She is an invaluable asset to the Annapolis Valley Regional School Board, as well as an active member of her community of Port Williams.

I do not know if you are aware of the mishandling of her medical case, but this is a woman who is fighting for her life due to years (YEARS!) of poor communication, doctor error, and questionable ethical practice. Due to not receiving the immediate treatment she required, she is now battling stage IIIC rectal cancer. As a young woman in her 40's, she has the health and attitude to beat this, but she will require the most aggressive and appropriate treatment available.

This treatment, known as FOLFOX, has been adopted as the best practice standard for chemotherapy among stage III rectal cancer patients in several provinces, including Ontario and BC as well as throughout the United States and Europe. It is considered by many provinces to be the best treatment. I am extremely concerned about the inferiority of NS treatment standards. I am more concerned about Robin, who once again, is denied the treatment she requires to live.

Nova Scotia needs to approve FOLFOX chemotherapy treatment for stage III rectal cancer. Lives depend on it.

Yours,

Allison McNeil

From: Kym Hume
To: Maureen MacDonald, Health Minister
Sent: Wednesday, November 10, 2010 4:30 PM
Subject: Treatment for colorectal cancer

Dear Minister MacDonald,

I am writing in support of my dear friend and colleague, Dr. Robin McGee (48), who has been undergoing cancer treatment for stage III rectal cancer. She has finished her initial treatment of radiation and chemo, had the surgery to remove the tumour, and is now taking oral chemo before undergoing surgery in the spring. The medical research in other parts of Canada and parts of the world, with regard to the appropriate treatment for both colon and rectal cancer, is clear. The agent FOLFOX has better results and is the recommended treatment for these cancers. Upon meeting with her oncologist, Robin and her husband were informed that she would not be receiving the agent FOLFOX in her chemo medication. (If she lived in Ontario or B.C., she would automatically have FOLFOX).

Her case is now before a medical board who are discussing whether this policy should change for all Nova Scotians with rectal cancer. Dr. McGee's case is urgent. She deserves the best treatment option available, and this must happen for her and other Nova Scotians who have or will have rectal cancer.

I urge you to intervene with the medical board who are presently discussing this case and make the decision to ensure that Robin McGee and all Nova Scotians have the same standard of cancer care as other provinces such as Ontario. FOLFOX must be authorized as a treatment for stage III rectal cancer. Robin and her family deserve to know that everything possible was done to help her battle this disease. She has so much to offer her family, friends, colleagues, and society. Please help her. She and her family desperately need your support right now.

Sincerely,

Kym Hume

From: Holly Gallagher
To: Maureen MacDonald, Health Minister
Sent: Friday, November 12, 2010 3:59 PM
Subject: FOLFOX treatment for rectal cancer

Good Afternoon Ms. MacDonald,

I am writing to you this afternoon in your capacity as the Minister of Health for Nova Scotia.

On November 9, 2010, Dr. Robin McGee wrote to you and her local MLA with an impassioned plea to authorize FOLFOX as a treatment for stage III rectal cancer patients in Nova Scotia. I am hoping by adding my voice to hers, as well as the other friends and family members who are contacting you on her behalf, that the best treatment option for stage III cancer patients will become available in this province.

I encourage you to review the information that Robin has provided. I understand that funding for health initiatives is limited. However, it is clear that FOLFOX is not only her best chance at survival, but it is ultimately the most cost-effective option.

Please bring the quality of NS healthcare on par with other provinces and consider the benefits of offering this treatment option to Robin and other stage III rectal cancer patients.

Sincerely,

Holly Gallagher

The day after I sent my email to him, my MLA Jim Morton calls me. He wants to clarify that the chemotherapy I am seeking is outside the formulary. He promises me that he will approach the Minister of Health and Wellness about this issue in the next few days. He remarks that he has received dozens of emails on my behalf in the past 24 hours.

"I cannot give you any promises," he says, "but I will look into this and get back to you. This might take some time to investigate."

I know I have to contact Dr. Dorreen to let him know what RCO and I have started. *Please don't be angry with me,* I pray as I feed the fax into the machine:

11 November, 2010

Hello Dr. Dorreen:

I am sending this fax as a "heads up" on some lobbying of the government I have done regarding extending provincial authorization of FOLFOX to stage III rectal cancer patients. I am also giving you my consent to speak to government officials about my case, in the event they contact you.

I emailed the Minister of Health Maureen MacDonald and my own MLA Jim Morton about the issue (see the text attached). Since then, the Minister of Health has received dozens of emails and letters from others in support of the issue, some supporting my case specifically.

Last night, I was called by my MLA Jim Morton, saying that he and the Minister of Health will be "looking into it."

Please consider this fax, and my signature below, to authorize you to release information about my case to any representative of government who may contact you to discuss it.

Perhaps government attention to my case will result in the funding required to prescribe FOLFOX treatment for me. Perhaps this attention will come too late for me. However, hopefully it will result in fostering dialogue between oncology experts and government policymakers to the benefit of your future patients.

Sincerely,

Robin McGee

Encouraged by my MLA's attention, I post further encouragements to the RCO community:

SEND THOSE EMAILS!
posted by Robin McGee, Wednesday, November 10, 2010, 5:15 PM

Thank you to everyone who emailed the Minister of Health on my behalf! It is possible that this effort is paying off! I just got a call from my MLA Jim Morton saying that he will ask her office to look into it. Possibly, this might mean I myself could get the treatment. Time is of the essence, as I would need to start FOLFOX treatment in the next 2 weeks.

Tell the Minister of Health, Maureen MacDonald, that you want Nova Scotians to have the same standard of cancer care as other provinces such as Ontario and that you want FOLFOX authorized as a treatment for stage III rectal cancer.

Thanks again to all!

I have started something. I have entered into an unknown, a place I have never been. It feels fragile and unstable, as if the ground beneath me might pitch and yaw like a sailboat. Inside, I feel a breathless hitch behind my ribs, like the sensation at the top of a roller coaster: dread and anticipation together. Trembling, I hold on to the supportive messages of the members of RCO, who salute my efforts despite the brink over which I hover.

Linda G < 11/10/2010 9:52 AM >

Again, God has you in the right place...your obedience and efforts to give a voice where there is none. It is comforting to see it from that larger perspective, knowing He's controlling all of it. It's so amazing to see the interconnectivity to all that happens. He's using you in the most incredible ways!!

Day after day, the RCO emails continue to pour into the office of Minister MacDonald. A veritable avalanche of letters.

From: Beth Robinson
To: Maureen MacDonald, Health Minister
Sent: Saturday, November 20, 2010 2:06 PM
Subject: Request that FOLFOX treatment be authorized for the treatment of Nova Scotia oncology patients diagnosed with rectal cancer

Dear Honourable Minister of Health:

I am writing to add my voice to the numerous requests that I know you've been receiving on behalf of a dear friend and colleague of mine, Dr. Robin McGee. After a series of apparent medical missteps, Robin was diagnosed last spring with stage III rectal cancer, and she is now fighting to regain her physical health and the quality of personal and professional life she previously enjoyed. In addition to being a well-loved daughter, sister, wife, mother, friend, colleague, and community member, Robin is an accomplished psychologist who has contributed much to the mental health and wellbeing of children, youth, and adults through her provision of services in community mental health, independent practice, and the public school system. It is through her keen scientific mind and accompanying competency in research that she has been able to mobilize during her illness and treatment. With her computer on her lap, and medical and research documents piled high around her on her sofa, Robin recently undertook the most poignant research project of her life: a quest to ascertain the optimal treatment for her late-stage diagnosis of rectal cancer. As the result of delving into medical protocols across Canada and the US, Robin has identified FOLFOX treatment as medically indicated for her type and stage of cancer, and the approach most likely to afford her the opportunity to watch her son grow to adulthood. It is a treatment offered to other patients in Canada and the US with rectal cancer in addition to those with a diagnosis of colon cancer (whom I understand to be the only potential FOLFOX treatment recipients at present in Nova Scotia).

I am contacting you in your role as Minister of Health in the fervent hope that you will revisit the current treatment protocol for Robin and other patients with rectal cancer, whose survival rate may well be increased by extending the opportunity to avail themselves of FOLFOX treatment.

Thank you for your consideration of this potentially lifesaving (for Robin and many others) request.

Beth Robinson, PhD, R. Psych.

From: Sarah Hergett
To: Maureen MacDonald, Health Minister
Sent: Monday, November 15, 2010 12:27 PM
Subject: cancer care treatment

Dear Minister MacDonald,

I am writing to you to support the request of a friend and colleague, Robin McGee. Robin has stage III rectal cancer. I understand there is a discrepancy in standard of care between NS and other provinces such as Ontario. Robin is looking for the FOLFOX treatment to be approved.

Robin has dedicated her life to helping others through her work as a psychologist. She is the hardest-working, most dedicated colleague I know. She has improved the lives of hundreds (if not more) children and families. I knew Robin first as a colleague at AVH Mental Health Services and have continued to work with her through her current role at the Annapolis Valley Regional School Board. I am advocating for a change in the treatment approved in NS. However, these changes take time, I understand. On a compassionate level, I would ask you to consider Robin's request more immediately. Robin has dedicated so much of herself to helping others through the public health care and educational system. She is an award-winning psychologist and invaluable employee and citizen. Her husband and son, as well as Robin, are anxious that she receive treatment that gives her the chance to carry on her work and her life—she's got lots left to do! As I am sure you are aware, Robin is at stage III due to physician(s) error. For this reason alone, I would hope the province would consider her case as a way to rectify a gross wrong that was done to her.

Thank you for taking the time to read and consider this request,

Sarah Hergett

From: Claire Wilson
To: Maureen MacDonald, Health Minister
Sent: Thursday, 18 November, 2010 11:50 PM
Subject: Authorization of FOLFOX for the treatment of rectal cancer

Dear Minister MacDonald,

I am writing to ask you to consider authorizing FOLFOX for the treatment of stage III rectal cancer, as is done in other provinces and the US. I am a friend of Robin McGee, who is a Kings County resident and stage IIIC rectal cancer patient. I understand that this cancer is curable, but the best practice treatment for it is not authorized in Nova Scotia.

It is alarming that Nova Scotia is falling below an internationally accepted best practice standard for the treatment of rectal cancer, putting residents' lives at risk. Robin is a wonderful person with a lively sense of humour and a marked intelligence. She is a friend, fellow soccer player, and gifted psychologist, as well as a loving and cherished wife and mother. Her diagnosis came as a shock to all of us who know her. I urge you to consider authorizing this treatment, which could save her life and the lives of other Nova Scotians with this kind of cancer.

Yours sincerely,

Claire Wilson

From: Tracy Tidgwell
To: Maureen MacDonald, Health Minister
Sent: Friday, November 19, 2010 10:58 AM
Subject: Greetings

Dear Maureen MacDonald,

I'm writing with deep concern for Nova Scotians who are living with and dying from colorectal cancer. As you know, right now, Nova Scotians are unable to access the best practice treatment for stage III colorectal cancer: FOLFOX. This chemotherapy is authorized and available to stage III colorectal cancer patients in several other Canadian provinces as well as in the US. I am asking you to help make FOLFOX authorized and available as a treatment for stage III rectal cancer *immediately*.

As you may also already know, Dr. Robin McGee, a stage IIIC rectal cancer patient in NS, needs this treatment *immediately*. Time is of the essence in her case. She needs to begin this treatment ASAP.

Please, PLEASE, help make FOLFOX authorized and available to Robin and to other colorectal cancer patients in NS *immediately*. You will help save lives.

Thank you,

Tracy Tidgwell

From: Tara Szuszkiewicz
To: Maureen MacDonald, Health Minister
Sent: Friday, November 19, 2010 12:35 PM
Subject: Calling all Nova Scotians

Dear Ms. MacDonald

Please consider authorizing FOLFOX treatment for the treatment of stage III rectal cancer, as is done in other provinces and the US. Time is of the essence for one of my colleagues, as I'm sure is the case for many patients across Nova Scotia who have been diagnosed with cancer.

I work in the NS health care system in Mental Health and pride myself on the fact that I provide evidence-based treatment for my patients. Why should Nova Scotian cancer treatment lag behind other provinces?

Dr. Tara Szuszkiewicz

From: Daphne Kennickell
To: Maureen MacDonald, Health Minister
Sent: Wednesday, November 10, 2010 7:08 AM
Subject: chemotherapy called FOLFOX

Dear Ms. MacDonald:

I am appealing to you for your help in authorizing a chemotherapy called FOLFOX in Nova Scotia for patients with stage III rectal cancer. My friend, Robin McGee, is currently undergoing treatment for stage IIIC rectal cancer, but is not undergoing the best-practice standard for chemotherapy. I understand it is authorized for colon cancer, but not rectal cancer. It seems to me there is a very small dividing line between the two. It seems to me that as tax-paying citizens, we should all be entitled to the best treatment for cancer. Cancer is cancer and patients should be entitled to the best treatments to secure a cure.

Best regards,

Daphne Kennickell

Some are from family:

From: Roberta E Clark
To: Maureen MacDonald, Health Minister
Sent: Wednesday, 10 November, 2010 9:33 AM
Subject: Appeal...

Dear Minister MacDonald,

I am writing today to beg, yes, beg you to carefully consider the issue of our province changing its stance on the health care issue of agreeing to give stage III rectal cancer patients the drug FOLFOX as their prescribed treatment, as is done in some other provinces and countries across the world with great success! How can one NOT agree that to provide the treatment that, though very harsh and demanding on one's body and endurance, gives a greater hope of cure and survival????? Would you not want that for your loved ones or for yourself?????????? I cannot understand why the decision is even debatable!

In the last 15 months, I personally have watched the death of a dear friend from colorectal cancer; knew the agony of a young friend's treatment and aftereffects of FOLFOX treatment in Ontario, and shared her joy that she has survived and is beginning to pick up the threads of her life thanks to that particular treatment; watched a sister grieve her daughter's cancer death; saw a cousin's wife die of lung cancer; saw my children's father suffer and die from throat cancer (incidentally, he went to Newfoundland and bought property there so at least he got the treatment he felt would give him hope); and then my daughter-in-law was diagnosed with stage III rectal cancer!

This has brought her life and her career to a standstill, as well as the lives of my son and my only grandson, who is just 15-years-old. Both extended families have endured great strain and showed much concern. My son is under too much stress to continue with his demanding and precise job as an engineer and is at his wife's side every moment. My precious grandson is coping with being in high school, adolescence, and the ongoing battle by his mother to try to increase her chances of being alive for him. He is overwhelmed by the enormity of this life-changing event in his young life. My daughter-in-law, herself, is courageous and selfless enough to be willing to face any and all the radical, often brutal, side effects of receiving FOLFOX...she should NOT be denied that chance, not under any law or budget issue. Oh, please, please, please give her that chance! This plea comes from my heart, which is broken because my dear brother died last week... of cancer!

Very sincerely yours,

Roberta E. Clark

From: Patricia McGee
To: Maureen MacDonald, Health Minister
Sent: Thursday, 19 November, 2010 12:36 AM
Subject: Robin McGee

Hello Ms. MacDonald:

Robin is a very precious niece. She really needs the best treatment possible. Please ask your Minister to consider her request for the most appropriate treatment, i.e., the FOLFOX treatment authorized for the treatment of stage III rectal cancer, as is done in other provinces and the United States.

Robin is a skilled professional who has much to offer to Nova Scotians as she practices her profession and contributes to her community—a valuable resident of Nova Scotia. You do not want to lose her.

Please consider her urgent request with all seriousness and compassion.

Thank you,

Patricia A McGee BScN MBA MDiv

Some of the letters were from other cancer survivors:

From: Shelley Hamilton
To: Maureen MacDonald, Health Minister
Sent: Tuesday, 16 November, 2010 11:06 AM
Subject: Sending to M. MacDonald

I am writing you, Minister MacDonald, to implore you to have the province change their stance on FOLFOX in stage III rectal cancer treatment. I am a Maritimer who has lived in Ontario for years and have worked here professionally as a singer and actor. Nova Scotia will always be my home. I come back regularly to work; but not since 2009, when I was diagnosed with aggressive stage III colon cancer.

I have had 60% of my bowel removed and have done 12 treatments of FOLFOX—the treatment used in Ontario, other provinces, the U.S, and Europe. When I was diagnosed, my husband and I were very proactive and have several connections in the medical field, so we were able to consult with many people and research treatment options, and from ALL our connections and research, (one of them being a Member of the Order of Canada who specializes in the field and is still on the Princess Margaret Hospital board), it is HIGHLY recommended that FOLFOX be used for aggressive stage III colon and rectal cancer. As difficult as the treatment was, I managed it well with help from friends and my medical support system here in Ontario.

I was saddened and frustrated to hear that a fellow fighter in the war in Nova Scotia, Robin McGee, is not able to receive this same treatment in Nova Scotia when it has been proven to have high success rates in fighting this disease. The system and the doctors that treated her before her diagnosis dropped the ball, and now in her stage III diagnosis, I feel that the system is letting her down AGAIN as well as others with this same stage III diagnosis. I implore you, and implore the province, to change your stance on treatment on stage III rectal cancer. Colorectal cancer is the silent killer in Canada and is the SECOND leading cause of cancer death in Canada. How is it that individuals facing such a silent killer—one that can be battled and won with correct care—are not given a fighting chance in my home province? This saddens me for good people like Robin and for others fighting this type of cancer right now.

I implore you, change this stance and allow a wonderful woman, wife, professor, and mother like Robin McGee, and others, a chance to still be with their families and loved ones. With cancer, it's not how or who...but WHEN. And if this cancer affected your loved ones or if it ever does, you WILL want this care in place to save their lives. Trust me, I am so thankful to have had this treatment, and as I heal, I can say..."I'm still here."

Creatively yours...

Shelley Hamilton

I see that several members of RCO members have contacted MLA Jim Morton directly, asking him to intervene on my behalf. His office responded to their requests.

From: Joan and Roger B
To: Jim Morton, MLA; Maureen MacDonald, Health Minister
Sent: Friday, November 19, 2010 6:59 PM
Subject: Robin McGee

Hello Minister MacDonald:

I am a friend of Robin McGee and request URGENT action on her behalf.

Thank you.

From: Jim Morton, MLA
To: Roger and Joan B
Sent: Saturday, 20 November, 2010 10:37 AM
Subject: Fw: Robin McGee

Hi Joan,

Thanks for copying me on this message. I want you to know that
I have spoken with Robin. I am also talking with officials in the
Department of Health and with the Minister about Robin's treat-
ment needs and will continue to help make this a matter of priority.

In the meantime, my thoughts are with Robin and Andrew and their
family during such a difficult time.

Jim

Some writers write for me personally. Some request FOLFOX
for all patients with node-positive rectal cancer. Some of the RCO
community get their friends, family, and colleagues to send emails
as well. In some schools, each member of the staff sends an email.

I am overwhelmed by the supportiveness of the responses, the
kind things that many say about me as they argue for my chance
at survival. Like many, I came home from work to my own home
routines; I had imagined myself as living my own quiet life. I had
no idea of the magnitude of my impact on others, of the degree of
attachment we shared. It hurts to reflect that it has taken cancer
and the threat of death to realize just how connected I am to my
community.

I am also moved by the genuine pain from which many are
writing: the loss of loved ones to this disease. One responder
describes to me how her email to the Minister described the anguish
of watching her brother die of stomach cancer, and her sickened
reaction after learning that Nova Scotia did not have best-practice
cancer treatment. If Nova Scotia fell behind other provinces with
my cancer, who is to say that they are not falling short in other
cancers? They had trusted the doctors when they told her brother

his protocol, but who is to say that he might not have lived if he had received another treatment used elsewhere? How could she ever trust cancer care in this province again?

Ordinary citizens are pouring out their hearts to a waiting government. *What will happen next?*

20

I DID NOT UNDERSTAND THE FLOW OF CANCER DRUG FUNDING in Nova Scotia. I learned it later, but at the time I did not realize its complexity.

Typically, any recommendation begins with an internal committee known as the Site-based Team. These are multidisciplinary teams that meet frequently to do case review, as well as to advise on practice issues. They are comprised of experts in oncology, radiation, surgery, imaging, and pathology. Teams tend to focus on specific cancers. For example, all gasterointestinal cancers are reviewed by one GI Site Team. Cancer Care Nova Scotia (CCNS), the branch of the government that facilitates cancer care, sends a representative to the meetings on a monthly or quarterly basis to discuss guidelines and policy. The frequency of Site-based Team meetings is determined by patient load as well as the "hotness" of the topics under discussion. With the guidance of CCNS, the Site-based Teams can propose the review of new cancer drugs that they learn of through their experiences and research.

The second step in the process is the Oncology Therapy Subcommittee. This body reviews the recommendations and the evidence for a drug. This Subcommittee is internal to the QEII. It is tasked with assessing the evidence for a chemotherapy, and if it passes there, of recommending review by the next level of committee, the Cancer Systemic Therapy Policy Committee or CSTPC.

The CSTPC is a 23-member committee comprised of representatives from the medical community as well as bureaucrats from the Department of Health and the various regions of the province. Also on board are an ethicist and a cancer survivor. In addition to reviewing the evidence for the recommendations made by the first two committees, it also evaluates the economics and ethics of these decisions. It reviews the feasibility of adopting specific chemotherapy regimens over the whole province.

Once the CSTPC approves a recommendation, it "advises" the government to consider the recommended treatment for formulary funding. However, the government alone formally decides if the drug will be funded. The government may choose not to adopt a recommended drug for cost reasons or because they have other priorities.

When a patient needs a treatment that is outside the formulary, an oncologist can make an application for the funding required to an internal body known as the Oncology Internal Review Committee. Where there are requests for "one off" treatments and no formal submission is in the works, decisions to allow or refuse individual requests are made by this committee. The general rule is that if more than two requests for a particular treatment are made and accepted, the expectation is that any further requests should go through the formal process.

What I did not know, but came to learn, was that other rectal cancer patients had appealed for Oxaliplatin treatment before me. In 2007, another stage IIIC patient had appealed for FOLFOX across several levels of administration and government. Refused due to the "lack of evidence," he chose to travel to New Brunswick for his treatment, undergoing great hardship in the process. Eighteen months before I came to him, Dr. Dorreen had submitted a request to the exemption committee for FOLFOX for someone else. That patient had also been turned down.

My case arose during a time of growing restlessness among Nova Scotian oncologists. They could see that the international community had left the issue in the dust—the FOLFOX standard had been adopted by almost all major cancer centres in the Western world. It became clearer to them a definitive clinical trial of its application to rectal cancer would never occur because it was already universally accepted and used worldwide. They knew that if direct evidence was required prior to approval, funding was doomed. Oncologists were impatient and unhappy with this state of affairs.

Into this state of tension and foment, my RCO supporters have raised the flag of public outcry.

....

The government responds at last. A message is left on my voicemail by Kathryn Morse, the assistant to Minister MacDonald. She acknowledges that their office has received many emails on my behalf and that she has been tasked with "looking into it."

So again, I call upon the RCO Community:

CALLING ALL NOVA SCOTIANS
posted by Robin McGee, Thursday, November 18, 2010, 8:30 PM

> Hey RCO:
>
> For those of you Nova Scotians who have not yet emailed the Minister of Health, now might be a good time to do so! I got a call from one of her assistants this morning who left a message, but has not returned my calls. Her message said that the Minister is aware of my situation because of all the emails she is getting on my behalf, and the assistant has been "asked to speak to me."
>
> Email Maureen MacDonald, Minister of Health, and tell her you want FOLFOX treatment authorized for the treatment of stage III rectal cancer, as is done in other provinces and the US. Tell her that time is of the essence in my case.
>
> Maybe then this assistant will get back to me.

The RCO Community responds vigorously. Not only do they continue to email the Minister's office, but they share their encouragement with me for the fight.

Margie N < 11/18/2010 9:20 PM >

Hey Robin,

I have sent my email so hopefully it is one of the many that is bombarding the Minister's office! Maybe they are calling you, prepared to say "uncle" by allowing the FOLFOX treatment—here's hoping!!

Pauline C < 11/19/2010 9:13 AM >

My email has been sent off to the Minister of Health. Keeping my fingers crossed.

Diane H < 11/19/2010 9:11 AM >

Awesome response from all the people who care about you. You bet I have emailed and will continue to email her.

Beth R < 11/20/2010 2:12 PM >

If all of the folks on your Lotsa Helping Hands mailing list contact Maureen MacDonald, she'll be inundated indeed! It's pretty hard to ignore an email avalanche!! Here's hoping that the collective imploring for reconsideration of protocol moves things quickly in your favour.

I dream about you often; it must be vicarious visiting.

Stay strong—you are now fighting for many others walking a similar path.

Linda G < 11/22/2010 9:33 AM >

That's fantastic news!! Your case is forcing a conversation that wouldn't be happening otherwise! And now it is time to step back and see how it unfolds...it all comes down to trust, doesn't it? Hard to come by, but for some situations, it is your only real option. Being a therapist, you know you can take someone only as far as they are willing to go, and giving them the tools to make the right choice is what you hope you impart. You are in my prayers, daily...I pray you feel His presence today. XXXOOOXXX

I post:

THE LATEST DEVELOPMENTS
posted by Robin McGee, Saturday, November 20, 2010, 10:45 AM

Hello RCO:

Yesterday I got a call from Kathryn Morse, executive assistant to the Minister of Health. She told me that they had staff researching my issue and that they wanted to talk to my oncologist. I had sent them his contact info, but apparently he is away. Once they speak to him, they will get back to me. Hopefully, they will have something to say by next week.

Now I have to pray that my conservative oncologist, who is head of the Department of Oncology, will grab the brass ring we have given him through our lobbying. Some doctors resent government attention to their cases. However, hopefully he will see this as an opportunity to open dialogue between oncology experts and government policymakers. Hopefully, he will see this as an opportunity to get funding for me and other patients to have what his colleagues can offer in other provinces. I sent him my consent to talk about my case with the government by fax last week, along with a "heads up" that we were lobbying. So now I have done all I can...I just have to wait.

I am feeling more fatigued lately. Are the meds kicking in, or am I worn out from the struggle? Still no side effects yet regarding my hands and feet.

TODAY is Austin's 16th birthday! We both woke him up this morning with a birthday song and a hug. He is busy with the production of *Cinderella* this weekend. He was an "assistant stage manager"—a prop guy—and he really enjoyed it. His true love is sound production, so he hopes to do work on some other play with that skill set. Anyone need a sound guy? He has asked for slow-cooked baked beans for his birthday supper. He must be a true Nova Scotian!

It is the day I am to hear back from Ms. Morse. I have not heard. I appeal through email:

Robin McGee < 11/23/2010 10:31 AM >

Hello Ms. Morse:

When we spoke last week, you suggested I contact you on Tuesday (today) if I had not heard back regarding whether I can access FOLFOX treatment. Do you have any news for me? I am sure you can appreciate the stress of waiting.

Kathryn A Morse < 11/23/2010 10:38 AM >

Yes, I'm sure you are under a tremendous amount of stress. Staff here are still trying to contact with Dr. Dorreen regarding this issue. I hope to have an update from them this afternoon or tomorrow.

I pray that Dr. Dorreen will support me and support the cause. I pray that the government will listen to him. I pray that all ears and hearts will open.

The phone rings, and it is a timely surprise.

21

THE CALL IS FROM MY FRIEND AND COLLEAGUE JUDY Kavanagh, a resource teacher. We have worked together for years, committed to helping the dozens of troubled children and youth in our common care. Her second husband Brian had died a lingering death from cancer only a few years before.

"I have news for you," Judy crows. "I think we have a new way to get this FOLFOX approved! My daughter is Katie McNeil. She is the niece of Stephen McNeil, Leader of the Liberal Party in Nova Scotia. I have talked to her about your situation, and she has contacted her uncle about it. Once the Liberals research it, they may be willing to raise it in the legislature! So tell your online group to send all the emails they sent to Maureen MacDonald to Diana Whalen, Liberal Health Critic, and that will set it all in motion!"

Within the hour, I receive a flurry of emails regarding my situation from members of the Liberal party as well as Katie herself:

From: Katie McNeil
To: Diana Whalen, MLA; Leo Glavine, MLA
Sent: Tuesday, 23 November, 2010, 12:50 PM
Subject: URGENT!! Authorize FOLFOX for stage III rectal cancer

Mrs. Whalen and Mr. Glavine,

My name is Katie McNeil, and I am the niece of Stephen McNeil. I am emailing you because an educator, Dr. Robin McGee, in my community in the Annapolis Valley is dying from stage III rectal cancer, but stage III rectal cancer IS CURABLE. With a chemotherapy treatment called FOLFOX, this cancer can be cured. "However, in Nova Scotia, FOLFOX is authorized for colon cancer, but not rectal cancer." We have this treatment in our province, we are treating people with it, but Dr. McGee is going to die if she doesn't receive the treatment.

Here is a copy of a letter she has sent to Maureen MacDonald and Jim Morton...Dr. McGee needs this treatment ASAP—if she waits much longer, it will be too late. We need your help!

Mr. Glavine, I am aware that you are not her MLA and you are not the Health Critic, but you are the closest Opposition MLA to her so I figured it couldn't hurt to let you know.

Katie McNeil < 11/23/2010 4:08 PM >

Dr. McGee,

You don't know me, but my mom is a colleague of yours, Judy Kavanagh. She told me about your illness. I lost my stepdad to cancer, and I just can't understand why the government is doing this.

My uncle is Stephen McNeil and I have been in touch with some of his colleagues: Leo Glavine, who's the Liberal MLA closest to you, and Diana Whalen, who's the Health Critic.

I'm forwarding some emails from me to Leo and vice versa. I don't know if this will help you at all, but I had to try.

Robin McGee < 11/23/2010 6:21 PM >

Thank you so much Katie!!! How can I ever thank you?

Kathryn Morse, executive assistant to the Minister of Health Maureen MacDonald, has called me, saying her staff is "looking into it." She promised to get back to me tomorrow at the latest. She says they are trying to reach my oncologist but have not heard back from him. If this drags on much longer, it will be too late for me, but never too late to raise the issue in the House of Assembly for the protection of other future patients.

Katie McNeil < 11/24/2010 7:36 AM >

Dr. McGee,

There's absolutely no need to thank me. I think our government is being ridiculous about this, and there's no sense having contacts if you're never going to use them!

I don't know if you know Leo Glavine at all, but he used to be a teacher and a principal in the Valley as well and he got back to me immediately when I emailed him.

I really hope Kathryn Morse gets back to you today and I really hope this does not drag on longer than necessary, especially since time is of the essence.

My thoughts and prayers are with you, and I'll do whatever you need from the Opposition side of government.

Judy K < 23/11/2010 3:55 PM >

Robin

This is what Katie sent me. Leo knows that there are hundreds of teachers who have sent letters to Maureen MacDonald.

Jude

------Original Message------

From: Leo Glavine
To: Katie McNeil
Sent: Tuesday, 23 November, 2010 1:16 PM
Subject: Excellent Request

Katie,

Diana sits next to me in the House and we have asked our Health researcher to prepare an urgent request to the Minister. We are asking for a quick response. If we do not have a positive response, we will take the issue to the floor of the Legislature.

Thank you for bringing this very important matter to our attention.

Regards,

Leo Glavine

What to do with this information? I am moved and perplexed at the same time. What if Opposition involvement makes the government dig in to a refusal posture? What if this turns into a political or even a media circus? But if the government is not moving forward, how else will this treatment be made available?

I appeal once more to Ms. Morse:

From: Robin McGee
To: Kathryn A Morse
Sent: Tuesday, 23 November, 2010 4:10 PM
Subject: Re: Cancer treatments

Hello again Ms. Morse:

A new development has just occurred. Just prior to getting your last email, I was contacted by a representative of the Liberal party of NS, asking me to send my information to the Liberal Health Critic so that she can raise it on the floor of the House. They learned of my plight from a friend.

I do not want to take this step before you have had a chance to address the situation. I suggest that your staff have Dr. Dorreen paged. His pager number can be obtained by calling the QEII.

She responds the next day:

Kathryn A Morse < 11/24/2010 2:54 PM >

Hi Dr. McGee:

No news. Still under discussion here. Hope to have something for you soon.

Now I have a decision to make. Do I give the government more time? Or do I throw my weight behind the Liberal effort to draw attention to the hole in our health care? I decide to give the government one more day to respond.

But Katie McNeil is a force to be reckoned with. She calls her Uncle Stephen to raise the issue with him in person.

Judy K < 11/23/2010 5:24 PM >

Robin:

Katie is in Winnipeg, and God love her, she called Uncle Stephen, Leo, and Diana as soon as I passed along your news. She is a McNeil (but has my good Kavanagh genes as well)—she loves the politics and all that goes with it.

Here's hoping they can put some pressure on. I wonder if everyone who emailed Maureen would resend the email to Stephen, Leo, or Diana.

Robin McGee < 11/23/2010 6:26 PM >

What an awesome girl!

Kathryn Morse, executive assistant to the Minister of Health, emailed today to say that her staff have not been able to reach my oncologist yet. She says she will get back to me tomorrow at the latest.

I will give her one more day. If nothing happens, I will call on "the community" to resend all their emails to Diana. I do not want the government to lock up with defensiveness, but if they are going to do that anyway—let's have at them!!!

I pass the day, and then the night. I hear nothing. Nothing is in my email inbox. I appeal once again to Ms. Morse, expressing my reluctance to turn the issue into a politically contentious one, but also expressing my resolve to move the issue forward this way if this is the only way I can do so.

Robin McGee < 11/24/2010 12:19 PM >

Hello Ms. Morse:

Do you have any news for me?

The Liberal Health Critic has taken an interest in this issue. They have suggested that it would help them if I encouraged all those who emailed the Minister to forward their emails to Diana Whalen.

I would hate for this issue to become a political circus, or for the government to become defensive about the current policy under attack from the Opposition. However, I need to pursue whatever means I can to help myself and others. I would like an opportunity to discuss this step with you before I take it. If I have not heard from you by the end of today, I must go ahead with it.

The day passes. I hear nothing.
That night, I call on the RCO Community once more.

NEW DEVELOPMENT: REQUEST TO FORWARD
posted by Robin McGee, Wednesday, November 24, 2010, 3:00 PM

Hello RCO:

The Liberal Health Critic Diana Whalen has taken an interest in my plight. She is considering raising it in the Nova Scotia Legislature. This may be the only way progress can be made.

She suggests that each of you who emailed Maureen MacDonald would forward your original email to her.

The government emailed today to say the matter is "under discussion"—they have no news for me.

Thanks to all for all your support!

Judy K < 11/24/2010 4:27 PM >

Robin

I've sent mine on to Diana, Stephen, and Leo. Best of luck. Katie asked about you today—she spoke to Stephen again last night and told him that this level of health care is unacceptable in NS and that he'd better kick ass—he's her uncle, so she can say stuff like that. This is what I sent:

Dear Minister MacDonald:

I implore your government to allow and pay for the FOLFOX treatment that is standard in most provinces to be put on the forefront of the NS budget and be immediately effective in our province.

NS should not be substandard to any other province in cancer care. We have a wonderful, productive, much-loved, and respected member of the AVRSB—Dr. Robin McGee, who needs this treatment to allow her to heal and come back to improve the lives of so many of our neediest children. She is invaluable to us and her family, and we need to offer her any chance for increased survival.

Please act quickly to ensure she can start this treatment immediately.

Judy Kavanagh
A Nova Scotian who has lost too many people to cancer.

....

As the days unfold, my smartphone keeps singing. RCO members are once again responding, copying me on their emails to Diana Whalen's office.

From: Sonya Major
To: Diana Whalen
Sent: Wednesday, 24 November, 2010 3:16 PM
Subject: FOLFOX treatment

Hello Diana—

I would like to have my voice added to those who are strongly encouraging our government to fund FOLFOX treatment for rectal cancer—a treatment that is available in other provinces. Quality of cancer care should not depend on which province you happen to reside in.

My friend, Robin McGee, and anyone else who is battling this brutal illness deserve the best treatments available.

Sonya Major, PhD

Beth Robinson < 11/24/10 4:15 PM >

Dear Liberal Health Critic Diana Whalen:

As per Robin McGee's suggestion, I am forwarding a copy of an email (it follows below) that I had previously sent to Maureen MacDonald. Thank you for becoming involved in exploring the feasibility of granting this potentially lifesaving request.

Beth Robinson, PhD, R. Psych.

Barbara Clow < 11/24/10 3:42 PM >

Dear Diana,

I am forwarding to you a copy of the email request I sent to Minister MacDonald. As you are my MLA, I would be most grateful if you would follow up on this issue on behalf of my dear friend Robin McGee. I would be glad as well to hear from you about progress on this concern.

Sincerely,

Barbara Clow

Each RCO community member who has written to Whalen's office has received a prompt reply:

From: Diana C Whalen
To: Barbara Clow
Sent: Thursday, 25 November 2010, 4:11 PM
Subject: Re: FW: Coverage and authorization for chemotherapy in Nova Scotia

Dear Barbara,

Thank you for contacting me about the cancer drug FOLFOX for the treatment of rectal cancer.

In the last two days, I have received many emails on behalf of Dr. Robin McGee. I am the Health Critic for the Liberal Party; in that capacity, I have raised the issue with our research staff to find out more about this situation.

We have contacted Cancer Care Nova Scotia to get their input as they are responsible for studying and recommending cancer care drugs.

Robin herself is waiting to hear back from the Minister of Health's executive assistant and I am going to find an opportunity to speak to Maureen Macdonald, the Health Minister, about this at the legislature.

I really appreciate hearing from so many colleagues and friends of Dr. McGee. We were not previously aware that this drug would be available in Ontario and elsewhere and we are looking into it right now.

Sincerely,

Diana Whalen

By the afternoon, I receive an email from Tracey Preeper, Director of Policy and Research for the Liberal Caucus.

Tracey Preeper < 11/25/2010 4:37 PM >

Good afternoon Dr. McGee!

On behalf of Diana Whalen, MLA and Liberal Health Critic, I am following up on the information you have sent and the many pleas of assistance and support received from your many friends. During your difficult journey, it must be comforting to know that you have so many great friends who have truly been exceptional in their advocacy for you.

I wanted to follow up to let you know that I have made contact with Cancer Care Nova Scotia and Diana is going to try and speak to the Minister of Health in the legislature about FOLFOX.

If you could do us a favour and let me know whether you hear from anyone from Cancer Care Nova Scotia, the Department of Health, or even your own specialist with a status as to the request for funding of FOLFOX for stage III rectal cancer, that would be a great help.

I will connect with you again on Monday and we will see whether any progress has been made, and if not, we will work on a Plan B.

Take care and we will chat soon!

Robin McGee < 11/25/2010 5:48 PM >

Thank you so much Tracey!

My last contact with the government was yesterday, when Kathryn Morse, executive assistant to the Minister of Health, responded to my email inquiry by saying that the issue was "under discussion." She had no other news for me.

I will most certainly keep you abreast of any communication I get from any official source about this issue.

I see my oncologist Dr. Mark Dorreen of the Cancer Care Centre at the QEII next Thursday, 2 December 2010. I have given

Dr. Dorreen consent to speak with you or any other government representative regarding my case.

Dr. Dorreen has presented my case to a special committee of oncologists at the Cancer Centre. This committee will decide if they can make a special exemption to provide FOLFOX treatment in my case. I have been told that the committee may support FOLFOX for my treatment from a medical perspective. However, they have "maxed out" their chemotherapy budget for this year; they may have to refuse me for lack of funds. There has been no word from this committee so far.

Yes, the support of my friends and my community has been comforting and encouraging. We are all very impressed with the prompt attention that you and Ms. Whalen have given my case and the issue. If we are successful in obtaining this treatment for Nova Scotians, the whole province will thank you.

The Liberals have joined the fray. They are in the thick of it, and so is the RCO community.

22

THE INTERNET CAN BECOME THE GAMBLING ADDICTION OF cancer patients. You go online, hoping to hit that jackpot of hopeful news and information. Each search is like pulling the handle on a slot machine. You watch the words roll up the screen hoping they will stop on a win. But what happens? A series of losses, each more devastating than the last, as the grim statistics come before you. You search again, thinking that the streak of "bad luck" must eventually end. Sometimes, you come across a tiny nugget of hope. But those only make you return relentlessly to the screen, miserable but driven. And what does it matter? The statistics one reads are based on great groups of people. But your own journey is your own—what does it matter if 30% of people survive your cancer if you are not in that lucky percentage? When you are dead, you are 100% dead.

Driven, I read. I read several surgery journals and book chapters about surgical approaches to rectal cancer. I read about lymph nodes. Rectal cancer patients can have lymph invasion in the "mesorectal" area, which is just outside the rectum, but they may also have invasion in the "lateral" area – which is further away in the groin. When the lateral nodes are invaded by cancer, the book explained, the prognosis is extremely grim. Crucial nerves surround these nodes. Surgery can destroy a person's urinary and sexual functioning. Western surgeons generally consider that area to be inoperable. Although Japanese surgeons have developed techniques for the removal of cancerous iliac nodes, research on outcomes show no improvement in survival. Patients with cancerous iliac nodes do not make it.

As I read, a new terror steals over me like a python on a branch, crushing something fragile. *Didn't my diagnostic imaging reports say something about the iliac node?* I go to the thickening binder where I carefully contained all my medical reports. I shuffle anxiously through the papers, finding Dr. McIntyre's initial assessment report. "There is a question," it reads, "of internal iliac node involvement which is obviously a bad prognosis." Frantically, I leaf forward to the diagnostic imaging reports.

There is no mistake. *Both* MRI and CT clearly describe a greatly oversized internal iliac lymph node considered "highly suspicious" for metastasis. The papers I am reading specify that a normal iliac node is about 5 mm in size. Nodes of 8 mm are concerning. My right internal iliac node was 1.1 cm—more than twice the normal size.

I slam down my binder and swing into my computer chair, punching on the internet. I know that I had four of nine lymph nodes from the mesorectal area that were positive for cancer—I remember that from the pathology report. *But what about this iliac node?*

With growing apprehension, I read papers on the survival chances of patients with both mesorectal and lateral node involvement. In a 2001 paper by Japanese surgeons, I read: "that the survival outcome of lateral node-positive patients having three or fewer nodes, including nodes involved in the mesorectum, had a 75% 5-year survival rate, whereas patients with four or more involved nodes had only a four percent survival rate."

I frantically flip through my binder until I get to the report from my surgery. *Maybe they took it out?* Scanning through the paragraphs, I can see no mention of the iliac node. The resident's report seems comprehensive to me, being several pages. *So what happened to it? If they did not take it out, is it still there? Do I still have cancer inside me? Inoperable cancer?*

As I sit in front of those lines, a new knowledge emerges like a submarine surfacing in an arctic wasteland. The news is clear, grim, and unequivocal: someone like me, with four positive mesorectal nodes and one positive lateral node, has *only a four percent chance of survival.*

Four percent.

....

Christmas is nearing. Austin is a bass in the Annapolis Valley Honour Choir, a choir of auditioned high school students from throughout the region. Justly famous for their quality and skill, they attract a huge audience for their annual Christmas concert. They are performing along with the breathtakingly gifted harpist duo Ardyth and Jennifer.

I go to the concert in fear and trembling. *Four percent.*

The choir sings a soulful song that calls upon God to "hold me, rock me." They sing, "I've got a home on the other side."

Four percent. My throat is closing over with grief. *This is my last Christmas.*

I try to train my mind to the ethereal and beautiful music, and I catch wisps of its aesthetic transcendence between the intrusive dread that chokes me, pulsing with sorrow with each beat of my leaden heart. *I must leave my family.* Each moment seems to sear me with its fragility. *I have so much unfinished.*

Each thought is crowded by others—each minute fraught with a thousand possibilities. Thoughts of acceptance chase thoughts of anger chase thoughts of fear chase thoughts of hope that I might be an exception. *Someone has to be in the four percent—why not me?* Between raising a foot to walk and putting it down again, between standing and sitting down again, there were myriads of impressions, a miasma of conflicting griefs and comforts. Hope blew in and out of my mind like snow on a windowsill. The fear becomes so great that it almost lost its meaning, as the numbness of despair overtakes my senses. I try to steady myself: I take my next breath, and then the breath after that.

When I walk out of the concert hall afterwards, I glimpse Dr. Three among the throngs of attendees. I wonder if he will ever understand the enormity of the pain caused by his conduct.

I am still waiting for the government to respond. There is no news. But believing that I have inoperable metastatic disease has made all things desolate.

23

I open my email and I see it. The government has rejected my plea.

Kathryn A Morse < 11/26/2010 2:36 PM >

Hello Dr. McGee.

The Minister has reviewed the information provided by staff and will not be making an exception to cover FOLFOX as you have requested. Nova Scotia has a well-established process to review funding for cancer therapies. That process includes input from clinical specialists as well as a large committee of stakeholders who consider evidence as well as ethical factors in making funding recommendations to government. The Minister respects that process and does not wish to provide a drug to one person that has not been recommended to be funded for others in similar situations. She regrets that her decision could not be more favourable.

Kathryn Morse
Executive Assistant to the Minister

So there it is.

I read this response without surprise, almost without emotion. A kind of numbness descends. My last hope is gone. I watch it disappear, as a shipwrecked person sees a distant unknowing vessel vanish over the horizon.

It was a long shot, I console myself. *Of course there has to be a rational approval process. Of course they were going to refuse you.*

I stand up from the computer and wander as if dazed to my backyard window.

Outside, the November winds are screaming around our house, lashing the trees and driving white wisps of snow before them.

I press my forehead against the cool windowpane. *You tried, at least you tried.*

The backyard of our house borders a farmer's field that stretches far into a rolling distance. My sister Debbie had recently visited me from her home in Newfoundland to attend a nearby Buddhist retreat. I had tied the colourful Buddhist prayer flags she had given me to my wire backyard fence. I see them now, snapping in the wind, straining towards me like dogs on a leash. *The prayers are blowing into the house,* I think bleakly. *If only prayers were enough.*

I return to the computer. I read the response again. Something is still not right. This answer is vague. It does not address whether the formal process will ever be initiated for the treatment. So the door was closed for me—that was clear. But what about others? I type a question.

Robin McGee < 11/26/2010 3:59 PM >

Hello Kathryn:

Of course I am deeply disappointed to hear this. I understand that the government will not consider my personal case. However, does your response imply that the government will not consider covering this therapy ever? Will FOLFOX for stage III rectal cancer be reviewed in the official process you describe? Or does the government consider this discussion closed?

Kathryn A Morse < 11/26/2010 5:04 PM >

Hello Robin.

I knew you would be disappointed and I feel badly about being the bearer of bad news. The discussion is not closed. FOLFOX may be reviewed for rectal cancer at some point in the future.

Robin McGee < 11/26/2010 5:20 PM >

Did you ever reach Dr. Dorreen?

Kathryn A Morse < 11/26/2010 5:26 PM >

We did.

Robin McGee < 11/26/2010 5:38 PM >

Are there plans to formally review this therapy?

But there is no response. *So they reached Dr. Dorreen,* I think sadly. *I wonder what he said.*

I follow up with my MLA:

From: Robin McGee
To: Jim Morton, MLA
Sent: Friday, November 26, 2010 4:21 PM
Subject: Fwd: Response re FOLFOX

Hello Jim:

I understand that they will not make an exception in my case—but does this response mean that the NDP government will not consider this therapy for review via the official funding review process? Will FOLFOX for stage III rectal cancer ever be considered? The lobbying taking place in our community for this issue was not just about me personally, but for the issue generally.

Jim Morton responds to my email by calling me. He has been tasked with the unenviable job of explaining to me the rationale for the government's rejection of my plea. He is good-natured and apologetic, but nonetheless clear.

"We talked about it," Jim says. "I met with the Minister about it shortly after getting your first email. We put a team on it, including a pharmacist. We had a meeting with me, the pharmacist, and the Minister, plus support staff. In the end, we decided that we just could not afford it. We have a treatment that works well now, the 5FU therapy, and the difference in the survival outcome was not significantly large enough to merit that expense right now." He reminds me that the government has recently extended the formulary to cover drugs related to macular degeneration; that had been a long-overdue but costly decision. The government may reconsider in the future, but only if the CSTPC were to formally recommend it.

I pass the discouraging news on to the Liberals.

From: Robin McGee
To: Tracey Preeper; Diana Whalen, MLA
Sent: Friday, 26 November, 2010 3:56 PM
Subject: Rejection

Hello Tracey:

This is the response I got from the government today. They seem to miss the point that we were seeking funding for FOLFOX for future patients, not just me. Does this response mean they will not review this therapy for funding ever?

I pass it on to the RCO community:

GOVERNMENT REFUSAL
posted by Robin McGee, Friday, November 26, 2010, 4:00 PM

Hello RCO:

The government has refused FOLFOX in my case and seem to reject the whole issue. I cannot tell if they will consider it ever, for anyone, through the review process described. Here is the text of the email I just received. I have passed it on to the Liberals.

But members of the RCO Community do not take the news lying down. Several bridle at the decision and are raring to fight further.

Alison L < 11/26/2010 4:43 PM >

Oh Robin,

I am SO sorry that they have made this very short-sighted decision. So...what is plan B???? Can we help with more lobbying? Keep your chin up.

Tracy T < 11/27/2010 1:55 AM >

Ugh. So disappointed to hear this, Robin. What's their damage??? Arrrgh!!!! Please let me know what more there is to be done.

Sarah H < 11/29/2010 4:10 PM >

I am so sorry to hear about the setback. Let's see what the Opposition has to say.

Thinking of you.

Beth R < 11/28/2010 5:01 PM >

I am disheartened to hear this. If there is a logical line of reasoning in the message below, it eludes me. One would anticipate that the process of engaging government in reflection on an earlier decision (in this case regarding FOLFOX) would begin with a request by an individual for revisitation of that earlier decision. This does not mean that the request is being made for that one person alone. We made it clear in our submissions that you were the primary reason for our interest in FOLFOX treatment, but we hoped that this consideration would be extended to others in similar situations. One only has to do a superficial online search of FOLFOX treatment to discover frequent reference to its appropriateness for "metastatic colorectal cancer," not just colon cancer. I wonder if the stakeholders referred to include individuals with colorectal cancer. I wonder also which "ethical factors" have been referenced in the message.

I wish in no way to downplay the seriousness of macular degeneration, but believe that the lobbying to seek provincial funding for its treatment should be seen as less of an imperative than consideration of treatments for life-and-death conditions, if government monies are limited.

Many RCO members step up their efforts to involve the Liberals in the quest to save me.

From: Barbara Clow
To: Diana Whalen
Sent: Tuesday, 30 November, 2010 12:02 PM
Subject: RE: FW: Coverage and authorization for chemotherapy in Nova Scotia

Hi Diana,

Thanks very much for getting back to me so promptly. I understand from Robin that she has now heard back from the Minister's assistant and the response was not positive. If you could follow up with Minister MacDonald, that would be great. Robin has a very small window of opportunity to receive this drug.

Surprisingly, the Liberals do not seem daunted at all by the refusal. Tracey Preeper and Diana Whalen continue to investigate the issue.

Tracey Preeper < 12/1/2010 3:30 PM >

Hi Robin!

I apologize for not getting back to you in a more timely manner.

I don't believe this response means they will not ever review this therapy...it simply means it is in a queue with a whole host of other therapies that are being considered. It is my understanding that Dr. Dorreen may be a member of the CSTPC committee, although membership on the list is not publicly available.

When our Health Critic, Diana Whalen, spoke to the Minister, she seemed to allude to FOLFOX being in the queue but would not commit to it being considered sooner (which Diana requested she do).

I understand from your earlier message that you have an appointment with Dr. Dorreen tomorrow. He may be able to shed some more light on the issue of FOLFOX and the review committee tomorrow. I further understand that you are still waiting to see whether the therapy could be provided to just you in the interim until FOLFOX is considered by the committee inside the Cancer Care Centre.

Do you think you will hear word on this request from Dr. Dorreen tomorrow?

In speaking with Diana, she indicated that she would like to help you first and then move to the broader issue of all others. However, she does not want to push the issue of whether you would be able to access treatment through the internal committee.

Diana also wanted me to ask you: if you don't hear anything back, would you like her to ask a question in the House of Assembly, which would involve using your name? What are your thoughts on this??

I call her back. "Yes," I tell Tracey firmly, "I am open to being discussed in the Nova Scotia Legislature."

When I hang up the phone, exhaustion reaches through me. I feel so stretched, pulled thin and fragile like a spider web. Is my weariness due to the prolonged suspense about this treatment? Or is this the creeping fatigue of Xeloda chemotherapy, finally coming to take me under? I wonder vaguely if media attention to the FOLFOX cause might derail my complaint to the College of Physicians and Surgeons. *So many battles.*

Sighing, I go to the back window again and look out at the fields. The prayer flags are beating the air in the bleak and frenzied wind.

Four percent.

I know that I will need those prayers when I see Dr. Dorreen tomorrow.

24

WE SIT IN THE EXAMINATION ROOM AT THE CANCER CENTRE, waiting to see Dr. Dorreen. *What had he told the government? Had I misjudged his support for FOLFOX in a case like mine? Had he told them there was no evidence for it? That the request was incorrect and presumptuous on my part?* I wonder how he will greet me. *Will he be furious with me over my lobbying? Will he tell me to butt out of the oncology business? Will he consider my efforts as critical of him, as trying to hijack my adjuvant therapy? Have I have gotten him in trouble?*

The door opens. Dr. Dorreen comes in toward me, beaming, his hand outstretched to shake mine.

"Well," he says jovially, "You have certainly been in the news around here!" He smiles so warmly and with such obvious pleasure that my concerns about his potential wrath vanish.

He settles into the chair before the computer screen in the small examination room.

"Did the government call you?" I ask, tentative.

"I was called by a pharmacist from the government. They asked if I would recommend FOLFOX in your case. I told them that yes, I *would* recommend it in your case. And that I would recommend that it be added to the formulary for cases like yours."

Relief goes through me like a reaching tide.

"So now we have plans afoot to approach the government to ask them to approve the use of FOLFOX for rectal cancer. That is in process now, and if it all can get done in the next few months, there is a chance you could receive it. I have written a submission for the various committees it must go through. Then it goes to the government for the ultimate decision."

"Months? Is there any chance that I could get it? Would it be too late?"

"If it were approved within the next few months, I would give it to you. Even if it was only for one cycle. Even that would benefit you. But we need to be realistic that it is very unlikely that it will be approved in time."

"I worried," I say, "that you might be mad at me for interfering."

He shrugs and smiles broadly. There is no mistaking his pleasure. "Oh, on the contrary, this is a wonderful development...we are all behind this here. Everyone agrees that it is time for this to happen—long past time." He pauses. "And we could not have done it without you," he adds amiably.

I breathe out in relief and breathe in with fear. *I have something else to ask him.*

"I have another question I need to review with you," I say, trying to contain the anxiety that distorts my voice. "My diagnostic MRI and CT showed that my right internal iliac node appeared to be involved. I don't think that node was removed during my surgery. The papers I am reading suggest that this is a very grim prognosis..."

His thick brows knit. "Didn't Dr. McIntyre tell you he gave you a curative resection?"

"Yes...or rather, I overheard him tell someone else," I say, suddenly doubtful. *Had I misunderstood a comment meant for another patient?*

"Of all the surgeons, he is the one I trust the most. If he said that he gave you a curative resection, then that is the case."

"The stuff I am reading says that Western surgeons do not remove the iliac node if it is in trouble. If he did not remove it, what does that mean?"

Dr. Dorreen snaps on the computer in front of him. "Let's look through his surgery report," he says, quickly scrolling through a series of electronic documents.

"I can tell you that it mentions removing a large node, but not one in the iliac area—only the area next to the rectum," I say. "The report was not written by him, but by a resident."

Dr. Dorreen swivels in the chair to face me. "If this is true," he says gravely, "then you have stage IV disease. You would be considered incurable. We should be doing something very different with your chemotherapy." He looks thoughtful and shakes his head. "But I do not think this is true."

"I had a CT done after the surgery—when I was in hospital for that obstruction. There is no mention of any enlarged node in that CT. But they were looking for an obstruction, so maybe they did not mention it."

Dr. Dorreen looks at me sceptically. "They are trained to describe anything they see. They did not miss it. Why would you think that health care professionals would miss something like that?"

It was my turn to look at him sceptically. "You have read my assessment story," I say flatly. "This is me you are talking to."

He swivels back to the computer. "Let's look at that CT together."

He punches at the keyboard. The CT images swim onto the screen. As he rolls the mouse down the desk, grey and black images swell and recede on the computer screen like the blossom of a monochromatic flower.

"Right here," he says, stopping. "Come and see."

He points at the screen. "This is where that node should be if it were involved. I do not see any evidence of it. See?"

I squint at the image, uncertain of what I am looking at. I feel my breath.

"You can call Dr. McIntyre to confirm what I am telling you if you still have questions," he continues, "but on the basis of the information we have, I think we should proceed with treatment as planned."

The enlarged iliac lymph node can no longer be seen? Behind my ribs, the slightest breeze stirs.

....

Later in the afternoon, Dr. McIntyre personally returns my phone call.

"You are right," says his authoritative voice. "People with iliac node involvement have a very bad prognosis. And you are right, when the iliac nodes are involved, we don't take them out. The morbidity is too high, and the survival rate doesn't change. But I do not think you are one of those people. When we went in during surgery, I examined all your organs, including that lateral lymph chain. We don't open that area up, but I ran my fingers over it to feel for anything amiss. There was nothing. It did not look involved to me... Now, we did find lymph problems in your mesorectal area, which we took out completely. Your surgery was very successful from my point of view. You are thin, so it was easy to do."

"So what might explain the enlargement of the iliac node on the MRI and CT?" I ask. My head is swimming. I try hard to focus on his words. *Listen, you must listen carefully to him. It can still come undone.*

"Lymph nodes can be reactive. Maybe it was enlarged for some other reason. Maybe it was an artifact of the images. Maybe you got down-staged by the radiation. But I was *in there*, and I just don't think this is an issue for you. Now, we should keep an eye on it. We will take more images closer to the time of your reversal surgery. Because if it comes back, well...someone might go after it."

His steadfastness is bracing. I lean into it.

"So my survival chances...?"

"Look," he says directly, "no one has any business telling you that you only have a four percent chance of survival. Your chances are 50%, like anyone else with nodal involvement."

....

Andrew and I drive home that drab, drear, slushy afternoon. I watch the trees on the 101 Highway flash by. Slowly, incrementally, I integrate the words of both doctors. Dr. McIntyre could not see a problem in the flesh, and Dr. Dorreen could not see a problem on the post-op CT. *Maybe, just maybe...*

It starts as a flush, a wash over me. A tender, fragile sensation like a trembling, warming me, opening me. I have not felt this feeling in many months. *Hope*, I realize. *I am feeling hope.*

We are listening to the soundtrack album *The Boat that Rocked*. A sunny song begins to play: the 1967 oldie "98.6," sung by The Bystanders—the title is a reference to normal body temperature. The lyrics and the upbeat tune express the joyous return to health of a grateful lover.

As the song reaches its cheerful crescendo, my heart expands suddenly. *I can see a future,* I realize with wonder. A vista of opportunities expands rapidly before my mind's eye: *I could get to raise my son. I could stay with Andrew. I could go back to work.*

A trembling gratitude steals over me, engulfing me. *I have a halfway chance at survival.*

....

I post the news to the RCO community:

MORE FOLFOX NEWS
posted by Robin McGee, Thursday, December 2, 2010, 5:30 PM

Greetings RCO:

Well, we met with the oncologist today. More of that anon. He told us that when he was called by the government, he told them that he recommended FOLFOX for my case. He also wrote a letter to them requesting extension of the formulary to cover FOLFOX for all stage III rectal cancer patients. Far from being mad at me for starting the lobbying, he seemed delighted. He said it was not too late for me to start it. He said it would be good for me to have it, even if it was only for a few cycles. If the government would act quickly to authorize it, he would give it to me, even if only for one cycle. However, we are all anticipating it might take months to authorize, and I understand Minister MacDonald is not inclined to move it up the queue for consideration. The Liberals have asked if they can raise my name in the Legislature, and I have given my permission for that. So kudos to all of you who raised your voices to call for this change—it did some good, if only to better motivate the oncology community to argue for it. Someone someday will have his or her life spared because of it. All of you feel free to keep badgering MacDonald—she can only ignore the public so much.

In other news, he and my surgeon were able to give me some important reassurance today. Before my operation, the CT scan and MRI indicated the possible involvement of a certain lymph node—the internal iliac node. This is a node that was not removed during surgery, as it is in a very difficult position. My surgeon assured me that he looked for it but could see no evidence of an oversized iliac node during the operation. He said that the image on the CT might have been influenced by the "shadow" of a nearby node that he did remove. (Imagine looking at a small ball in front of a bigger ball—the photograph would make the small ball look bigger). My oncologist pulled up the CT scan I had taken after my obstruction; scrolling through the CT, he could find no evidence of the problem. So both of them think that it is not an issue. So guess what everyone? It was a GOOD thing that I had that bowel obstruction, as it gave us a postoperative CT to look at. The Lord works in mysterious ways.

...And I cannot express how much of a relief it is to learn this. All week, I have been burdened and haunted by literature that said that people with iliac node involvement only have a four percent chance of survival. All week, I have been terrorized and choked up by that statistic. It is funny to say it, but when they reminded me that my chances were more like 50-50, I felt relief and joy. How strange cancerland is! If someone told me a year ago that I had only a 50% chance of survival, I would have been devastated; but today, I hear that news as wonderful and hopeful.

ROBIN McGEE

25

It takes me some time to find out what had happened within the halls of the government. I piece the story together over time.

When each RCO member hit "send" on their personal missives, the emails on my behalf sped through the ether towards the public mailbox of the Minister of Health and Wellness. When they arrived, a complex government machine was engaged.

Each email is read by a special correspondence clerk at the Department of Health and Wellness. Each one is printed off and put into a binder—a thick binder—for the Minister to read. Health Minister Maureen MacDonald is famously conscientious about such letters and makes it her practice to read every one of them. The clerks also direct each email to their counterparts in the government department deemed most appropriate to field the question posed by the public. In my case, each email is copied to the Pharmaceutical Services branch. There, special correspondence clerks print off each email to develop their own comprehensive binder.

My MLA Jim Morton was as good as his word. Within days of my email to them, he had met personally with Minister MacDonald. They discussed the need for expert opinion to guide their discussion and arranged a joint meeting with Judy McPhee, Executive Director of Pharmaceutical Services for the province. In her government role, McPhee could be considered the province's top pharmacist.

McPhee met with both politicians, explaining to them the typical process by which cancer drugs are funded, as well as the history of Oxaliplatin in Nova Scotia. Together, they determined that an exception ought not to be made in my case. A clerk was commissioned to craft a response to me and to all my supporters.

The decision in my individual case had been made; from a politician's perspective, there was no need to take matters further.

In government, the politicians may change roles, but the senior civil servants do not. McPhee had been in her role with several previous governments; she had seen politicians ask for exceptions on behalf of their friends and constituents. A firm believer in the methodical and due process by which cancer drugs should be approved, she was understandably opposed to treating my case as a "one off" exception. She knew that FOLFOX had been approved for colon cancer as well as metastatic colorectal cancer. However, she also knew that the relevant committees had not examined the question of FOLFOX for rectal cancer. She knew that the government did not have a defensible answer to the questions currently raised by the public and the Opposition.

So McPhee picked up the phone. She made a phone call to Mark Dorreen—a pivotal phone call. Aware that I had given him consent to speak to the government, she specifically asked him if he recommended FOLFOX therapy in my case.

Yes, he told her. Yes, I would. Yes, I do.

The two of them discussed the history of FOLFOX. Why had it not been put forward for approval for curable rectal cancer, if he and other oncologists supported its use? Reminded about the lack of studies specific to rectal cancer, she told him that the government would look favourably upon it if he will put the drug through the formal review process for a recommendation on whether to fund.

For Dr. Dorreen, this was the encouragement he needed. Previously, such an initiative seemed doomed by the "evidence-limited" approach to drug funding adopted by the province. McPhee urged him to push the recommendation through the various committees quickly. She knew that citizens would demand an answer:

why was this treatment unavailable in Nova Scotia when it was the status quo throughout the rest of the Western world? Only an expert evaluation could answer them.

Dr. Dorreen and Judy McPhee had both been members of the Cancer Systemic Therapy Policy Committee since its inception in 2006. They both had been present when FOLFOX was recommended for colon cancer in 2007. But they both had another experience in common: as CSTPC members, they had seen a CSTPC decision overpowered by a political agenda and public pressure.

In 2007, two citizen petitions were tabled in the Nova Scotia Legislature, lobbying for funding for the cancer drug Avastin. Jim Connors, a Dartmouth lawyer and one-time president of the Nova Scotia Progressive Conservative party, collected thousands of signatures on a petition requesting formulary support for Avastin. A second petition was submitted by a 71-year-old woman whose son had spent thousands on Avastin treatments. Asked to review the evidence for Avastin, the CSTPC twice decided against recommending it. However, the public and media pressure continued unabated.

Jim Connors died of colorectal cancer in April 2008. Only a few weeks later, the provincial budget was tabled in the legislature. In his budget speech, the then-PC Finance Minister made the unexpected announcement that Avastin would be fully funded. The Deputy Health Minister followed with a media statement that the decision to fund Avastin had been made suddenly and "strictly for compassionate reasons." She acknowledged that the decision for funding had been made despite the CSTPCs recommendation against it.

Members of the CTSTPC were surprised and dismayed by the announcement. The Minister met with the disheartened committee to assure them that their work was not futile and that their opinions were valued and respected. The decision to fund Avastin had been a political one, made in response to the public and media demands.

So both Judy McPhee and Dr. Dorreen had seen firsthand what public pressure could do. Political commotion can wrest control of cancer drug funding out of the hands of experts and spin it into the arena of legislature shouting matches and media circuses. Both of them were committed to the integrity of the formal process. Because the political iron was hot, they both knew that the matter of FOLFOX had to be handled judiciously and *promptly*. They agreed that Dr. Dorreen would initiate the formal review process right away.

Dr. Dorreen prepared a submission summarizing the three- and six- year results from the MOSAIC trial, illustrating clearly the compelling data on improved survival for colon cancer patients. His document stated that almost all major cancer centres in North America, Western Europe, Australia, and New Zealand agreed that FOLFOX is an acceptable adjuvant chemotherapy option in node-positive rectal cancer. He made it clear that because of its universal acceptance in worldwide practice, a definitive clinical trial specific to patients with rectal cancer would never be carried out.

His first step would be to present the recommendation to his colleagues on the GI Site Team, hopefully before Christmas. Assuming the recommendation would pass, the next step would be the Oncology Review Subcommittee when that body met in January. If the experts agreed there was scientific merit to the recommendation, it would go before the CSTPC in the spring. Yet even if the CSTPC advised the government to extend the formulary to fund the treatment, the final decision would be made by the Department of Health and Wellness. Ultimately, the government would decide whether and when funding for FOLFOX for rectal cancer would occur, based on their priorities and budget concerns. There was a long road ahead.

....

I do not fully understand what the complexity of the process on which Dr. Dorreen has embarked. But emboldened by his confidence in the formal process, I try again to push for FOLFOX treatment:

Robin McGee < 12/3/2010 9:36 AM >

Dear Ms. Morse and Minister MacDonald:

I am emailing to update you. I saw my oncologist Dr. Dorreen yesterday. Dr. Dorreen is head of the Department of Oncology at the QEII. He told me that he told the DHW pharmacist who contacted him that he recommended FOLFOX in my case. He also said that he has written a letter arguing for the extension of FOLFOX to rectal cancer patients to the Cancer Systemic Therapy Policy Committee.

He says that it is not too late, from a medical perspective, for me to get this treatment. If the government were to bump consideration for FOLFOX up the queue and authorize it promptly, he would give it to me as soon as possible. It would do me good to get it even for one cycle. I have a window of about three months to get it.

If I were to pay out of pocket for a treatment that was eventually authorized, would there be any chance of recovering my costs from the government?

From: Kathryn A Morse
To: Robin McGee
Sent: Friday, 10 December, 2010 1:27 PM
Subject: Re: New information

Hello Dr. McGee—

Thank you for the update regarding Dr. Dorreen's treatment recommendation and his referral of the funding issue to the Cancer Systemic Therapy Policy Committee. If FOLFOX is recommended by the committee and accepted by the Department of Health, funding is provided on a go-forward basis. There is no retroactive payment policy in place for chemotherapy received prior to the review process being completed and funding approved. This is consistent with the way we fund other treatments and procedures.

I'm sorry I cannot assist you further in this matter and wish you the best in the treatments you pursue.

Kathryn Morse
Executive Assistant to the Minister of Health

When I receive the formal letter of rejection from the Minister herself, I post it to RCO:

MINISTER REPLIES
posted by Robin McGee, Sunday, December 12, 2010, 10:30 AM

Hello RCO:

Here is the response I finally got from Minister MacDonald. I am puzzled by it, because she says no one has asked for FOLFOX to be considered by the government committee—my oncologist, who is a member of that committee, has told me he has given them a written submission to the CSTPC requesting it. Also, she received several dozen emails from all of you raising the question. I will send this to the Liberals, for what it is worth.

From: Health Minister
To: Robin McGee
Sent: Friday, 10 December, 2010 3:29 PM
Subject: Re: Authorizing FOLFOX for stage III rectal cancer M1650

Dear Dr. McGee:

Thank you for your email of November 9, 2010, regarding funding for the chemotherapy regimen FOLFOX as adjuvant therapy in the treatment of rectal cancer. I am very sorry to hear about your diagnosis and appreciate that you have brought your situation to my attention.

As I am sure you are well aware, decisions regarding the funding of cancer therapies are very serious and a very important aspect of our health care system. That is why, in 2006, the Cancer Systemic Therapy Policy Committee (CSTPC) was formed in Nova

Scotia to assist district health authorities in dealing with increasing costs associated with new cancer therapies and the difficult funding decisions that need to be made.

The CSTPC is a 23-member provincial committee with representation from a wide range of stakeholders including cancer specialists, district health authorities, representatives of Cancer Care Nova Scotia, a medical ethicist, the public, and cancer survivors. The committee uses a unique framework which considers clinical evidence and economics as well as ethical considerations in making recommendations to the Department of Health regarding which medications should be funded. Approved therapies are funded through the new cancer drug fund, which has infused approximately 10 million additional dollars into cancer treatment in the province since 2006. More information on CSTPC is available at http://www.gov.ns.ca/health/cancer_drugs/.

Cancer specialists at the hospital level assess the clinical benefit and costs associated with each new therapy and determine if it should be reviewed for funding by the CSTPC. To date, funding for FOLFOX therapy as adjuvant therapy in rectal cancer has not been brought forward to be reviewed by this committee for funding.

I respect and value the difficult work of the CSTPC greatly and therefore FOLFOX use in rectal cancer would need to be reviewed and recommended by CSTPC before new funding could be considered through the new cancer drug fund. This is consistent with our standard that all new therapies must be reviewed by an expert advisory committee. It is also fair to patients who are waiting for funding of other cancer or non-cancer related therapies that are going through the usual review process.

I regret that I am not able to approve funding for this therapy at this time and understand that this situation will be far from satisfactory to you. While funding cannot be approved through the new cancer drug fund, this does not preclude the hospital from assessing your request through their own non-formulary process.

Thank you again for bringing this matter to my attention. Again, I am sorry my response could not be more positive at this time.

Yours truly,

Original Signed By
Maureen MacDonald
Minister

....

I am packing for the holidays. Before I begin, I fax the Minister's letter to Dr. Dorreen:

13 Dec 2010

Hello Dr. Dorreen:

Here is Minister MacDonald's reply. I am puzzled by her statement that no one has brought the issue to the Cancer Systemic Therapy Policy Committee, given that you have written to them. She also says that the lack of funding "does not preclude the hospital from assessing your request through their own non-formulary process."

I am longing to see my parents and family in Ottawa. *Will this be the last time I ever see them?* The clothes feel heavy as I lift them into the suitcase.

I mull over the correspondence I have sent and received. *It's all over.* I have come to the end of all options. There is no further hope for me for this treatment, and, it seems, for other future patients. *I cannot do any more.*

The phone rings. Andrew picks it up, and his face visibly whitens. He holds the phone out to me. "It is Dr. Dorreen himself," he whispers urgently.

In the seconds it takes to cross the room, my heart starts to pound. *Why was my oncologist calling me personally?* He never did that—only nurses ever returned calls. With each step, my appre-hension mounts as different scenarios beat across my brain: *the node has come back, the disease has upstaged, my chemotherapy is failing,* all in a wave. I take the receiver, my throat full of the grief-filled thought that I will not see my parents this Christmas after all.

Holding it steady, I take a deep breath. "Hello?"

"This is Mark Dorreen," says his resonant voice. "I just read your fax, and I wanted to call to clarify that my submission has not gone to the Cancer Systemic Therapy Policy Committee yet. It has made it through the first committee, the GI site team, but it has to go through another internal oncology committee here first."

He is not calling with bad news. The pounding pulse in my ears recedes slightly. "When will that happen?"

"The plan is for January. I do not anticipate any problems with that. Once it has passed our internal committee, then we will write a formal recommendation to the Systemic Committee. I wanted to clarify that with you, so that you understand where things are right now."

Dizzy with relief, I sit down on the edge of my bed. My hands are trembling. I press the phone firmly against my ear. "So you are meeting with other oncologists in January to vote on whether to submit to the Systemic Committee? And after that the submission goes forward? In January?"

"That's right. We are all behind it here, so I see it as a shoe-in. I get the feeling that the government wants us to recommend it. They *want* to support it. We want to seize that opportunity."

"Dr. Dorreen?"

"Yes?"

"Have a Merry Christmas."

He chuckles. "And the same to you."

26

I AM UNAWARE OF IT, AS I AM UNAWARE OF BREATHING. BUT another process is ongoing underneath the surface of my troubled life. I will learn later all that transpired while I struggled.

When the RCO emails arrive at the office of Diana Whalen, Liberal Health Critic, another machinery was engaged.

Alerted to my case by Katie McNeil, Stephen's niece, Whalen and Preeper were ready. As each RCO email arrived, they carefully reviewed each one. They were impressed: *each letter was unique*. Politicians are used to getting advocacy letters that read like formula. So many causes employ a "cut and paste" approach to email, in which all senders use the same content. But in my case, each letter shared unique details about the sender and about me. Individually crafted letters carry more political weight than cookie-cutter ones. Diana Whalen knew this. Moreover, she knew that the Minister knew it too.

If a politician receives even five letters from citizens asking for change, he or she is compelled to respond. Whalen's office received over 40 such emails on my behalf and on behalf of the issue of FOLFOX funding. The Liberals were aware that these emails represented only a small subset of those sent to Minister MacDonald.

Moved by my plight, Whalen reflected that such a dreadful situation could happen to anyone. She imagined what it would be like if she or a member of her family were in my circumstances. Well acquainted with the ways in which Nova Scotia fell behind other provinces in basic health care, she knew how hard my struggle had been. She had been an active patient advocate during the recent debate on macular degeneration. She had spearheaded initiatives to fund early intervention for children with autism. In her view, the government's response to me was disingenuous, as they did indeed know that Dr. Dorreen was striving to bring the treatment forward. She was concerned by the inherent unfairness of directing deprived cancer patients to the internal exception committee. Because the exception budget is so readily exhausted, only those patients who fell sick early in a budget year stood a chance. Although she supported and respected the formal process by which cancer drugs are approved, she nonetheless carefully considered how she might expedite things, both for me and for the process.

Tracey Preeper launched into her own research on FOLFOX. She contacted Cancer Care Nova Scotia to learn about its history in Nova Scotia and in other provinces. A cursory review taught her that FOLFOX is ubiquitously used as a standard of care treatment for node-positive rectal cancer in all Western nations, as well as in Ontario and British Columbia. She wrote to Dr. Dorreen to ask him specifically about the status of the recommendation within the formal approval process as well as the dates of the committee meetings.

From: Tracey Preeper
To: Robin McGee
Sent: Friday, 17 December, 2010 2:45 PM
Subject: Re: More info on MacDonald reply

Hi Dr. McGee!

Sorry it has taken me so long to get back to you. I was able to speak to Diana today with regard to your situation and here is what we will try to do next. Diana is going to send a letter to the Minister indicating that she is aware the extension will be brought forward to the CSTPC in January and to request that should there be a favourable response (which sounds like might be the case from Dr. Dorreen) that consideration be given by the Minister to provide the financial resources to fund the drug immediately. While we are not in the position to overrule the decision of the CSTPC, we can put pressure to bear on those who provide the financial resources to implement these decisions.

Has there been any word on the internal hospital committee and whether they had any financial capacity to provide funding in the interim? Even if you were able to start the drug until government makes their decision, pending a positive outcome from the Committee, that would be a help.

I apologize for asking more questions than providing solutions. However, please know that we are trying every avenue on your (and ultimately others' behalf) and hope we will have some better news in the days and weeks ahead.

From: Robin McGee
To: Tracey Preeper
Sent: Saturday, 18 December, 2010 12:40 PM
Subject: Re: More info on MacDonald reply

Hi Tracey:

All I know is what Dr. Dorreen told me: that he plans to make a submission to CSTPC in the New Year, but that first the submission must be reviewed by an internal oncology committee. I do not know of any of the dates for these committee meetings. Meanwhile, he has told me that the internal "exception to the formulary committee" is unwilling to fund FOLFOX for me because they are already way over their chemotherapy budget for this year, and funding me would mean taking the money from other hospital programs. I have asked if I can pay for the treatment myself (approximately $10,000), but have been told no—this would appear too much like a two-tier system. I understand some provinces, such as Ontario, allow patients to pay for treatments in situations like mine.

The Liberals knew that CSTPC approval was not enough. Even if the CSTPC approved FOLFOX in a timely way, this did not mean that the government would make funding available promptly. Governments can accept the recommendation of an expert committee, but let their own formal approval languish. Even when governments formally approve a drug, this is no guarantee of patient access: governments can phase in an approved treatment slowly and incrementally. Whalen knew that she needed to find a way that would get FOLFOX fully and promptly funded.

The NS Legislature was scheduled to sit in April of 2011. Typically, prior to coming into session, the governing party reviews issues in anticipation of those the Opposition will raise. Regarding FOLFOX, both sides of the House knew that the subject would be raised on the floor of the legislature if the funding issue was not resolved before April.

So Whalen sent a letter to the Minister. By doing so, she was implicitly warning the government that the timeline for FOLFOX approval was under Opposition scrutiny. She was putting them "on notice" that the Liberals were watching.

Both sides of the House knew how causes are fought. If a treatment was unfunded, it was not uncommon for the Opposition party to find a celebrity victim and bring that person to the legislature gallery. The Opposition would demand that an embarrassed Minister refuse the patient "to their face." Invariably, the media would pick up on these human-interest stories, and the appalling story of the patient would be spread across the media. Whalen knew that Minister MacDonald knew these strategies. When the NDP were in opposition, they often brought busloads of victims to the legislature. I had all the right features: a young professional, felled in her 40s by cancer and atrocious medical care, begging for a potentially life-saving cancer therapy available everywhere but Nova Scotia. Any government who refused to address the issues represented by such a case was inviting singularly bad press.

It served the Liberals well that the RCO emails conveyed such unique information regarding my case. Using the details of my story, they were able to convey to the Minister that I would make a dangerous celebrity patient.

Tracey Preeper < 1/4/2011 11:43 AM >

I am attaching a letter Diana sent to the Minister of Health prior to the Christmas break for your records. The purpose of this letter was to have the Minister contemplate a decision of funding in advance of the Committee meeting so that funding approval from the Department would occur more quickly.

I did attempt to make contact with Dr. Dorreen prior to Christmas and subsequently received a response in letter form in today's mail (January 4, 2011). Basically, his letter confirmed what we already know...that we must now wait until the subcommittee and the formal committee meet and make a decision.

We will keep in touch. I am out of country for the next couple of weeks. In the meantime, keep in touch with Diana at her email address.

And the letter was attached:

22 December 2010

Honourable Maureen MacDonald
Minister of Health
4th Floor, Joseph Howe Building
1690 Hollis Street
P.O. Box 488
Halifax, NS B3J 2R8

Dear Maureen:

I am writing you today on behalf of Dr. Robin McGee whom I understand has been in contact with you directly with regard to her personal situation.

As you are more than aware, Dr. McGee is battling stage III rectal cancer. For Dr. McGee, time is of the essence as her ability to access the FOLFOX treatment within the next couple of months will increase her odds of survival. This particular situation has been made more tragic by the fact that an improper diagnosis, despite Dr. McGee's own personal efforts to have her symptoms addressed, has further reduced her chances of survival. Time is obviously of the essence.

In your response to Dr. McGee's email request on November 9, 2010 received by her on December 10, 2010, you indicated she should approach the hospital with a request for funding through their non-formulary process. She has done so and has been told that they have exceeded the chemotherapy budget for this year and a positive response to her request would mean taking monies from other hospital programs.

She has also offered to pay for her first treatment herself (with no expectation of reimbursement) while waiting for the Cancer Systemic Therapy Policy Committee to meet and make a recommendation on FOLFOX for rectal cancer. This offer was denied as this would have the appearances of a two-tiered system. While there are several instances where private insurance covers treatment in-province not yet publicly funded (Avastin for colorectal cancer comes immediately to mind), I gather an offer of self-insurance is viewed somewhat differently.

The purpose of my contact today is to remind you of the urgency and a need for a timely response in the case of Dr. McGee.

I understand the Cancer Systemic Therapy Policy Committee will be meeting in January and will likely consider a recommendation on FOLFOX as a treatment option for stage III rectal cancer. While none of us can predict the outcome of these deliberations, I humbly request you consider Dr. McGee's personal circumstances and ensure there is a timely response from the Department should a favourable recommendation be forwarded by the Committee to the Department for funding in January.

Please accept my wishes for a wonderful holiday season!

Sincerely,

Diana Whalen, MLA
Liberal Health Critic

I respond gratefully, even as I know that the chances of my getting the treatment have receded beyond the point of no return. I have only three months left.

Robin McGee < 1/4/2010 1:26 PM >

God bless you Tracey and Diana for all your wonderful efforts on my behalf!

We have all done as much as we can now. Now we wait. Whatever the outcome, I will be eternally grateful to you both for your advocacy. I will certainly be in touch if I learn anything.

On 26 January 2011, the Oncology Therapy Subcommittee met. This committee, the second in the formal process, considers the scientific merit of each submission. Dr. Dorreen presented the case for FOLFOX. Despite the lack of randomized control trials for rectal cancer, all were in agreement that the results for colon cancer were utterly convincing. This committee voted in favour of the proposal. They recommended that the proposed guideline be put forward to the Cancer Systemic Therapy Policy Committee.

And now everybody waits.

27

IN THE ARENAS OF GOVERNMENT AND CANCER CARE, EVERY-
one is waiting to see what will happen to FOLFOX funding.
Meanwhile, our own lonely struggles continue.

Andrew has a growth on his temple. I am with him when he
shows it to our family physician Dr. Good.

"It could be one of several things," Adam says. "A cyst, a scar, or
a cancer."

See? I think. *See how easy that is, doctors? All you have to do is list
cancer as one of possible causes. This is how a REAL physician handles
that situation.*

"I will send an urgent request today for a consult from a dermatologist," Adam says. "You should hear within two weeks."

But we do not hear. Andrew's repeated calls to the specialist's
office go unreturned. When he finally gets through, he is told that
it is office policy that only the calls of patients are returned: he is
considered a non-patient. It took *another* referral from Dr. Good to
become one.

When the dermatologist sees Andrew, he examines his temple
carefully. He wonders if it is a squamous cell cancer—the same
cancer Andrew's father has just died of. He schedules a surgery in
January to remove the growth. We will have to endure the holidays
not knowing if we both have cancer.

Each night, we lie awake, staring at the ceiling. Cancer has a
way of waking you up—that is not a metaphor. It literally wakes

you, every night. Thoughts and fears and phantasms that stay away during daylight come crowding in during the small hours of the night.

How could we both have cancer? We had known couples where both parents were afflicted. *What if we both die? What would happen to our son?*

Remorselessly, cancer forces us to confront the anguished vision of such a future. *Where would Austin go at Christmas time when he was in university? Who would look after him, if he became sick or injured? Who would be there to celebrate with him when he graduated?* The thought of our only child all alone in the world is an anticipatory grief of unbearable magnitude. It is a monster's maw we both look down. Between us, the relentlessness of our terror pushes us into a state of suspension. We can endure it with only one sustaining reflection: *we are not both dead today.*

From Ottawa, I call the Cancer Centre for my monthly check-in. I describe to the nurse the drilling pain I am experiencing where I once had a rectum. She encourages me to take it up with Dr. McIntyre.

"It couldn't be a recurrence, could it?" I beseech her. "So soon? My surgery was only three months ago."

Her reply is bloodfreezing: "Cancer can do anything," she answers.

Under the bombardment of chronic threat, the fear fills every tedious minute. Waiting for the Sword of Damocles to drop—waiting for the test results or, worse, when you have them and they are disappointing—you are catapulted into a state of apprehension so intense and all-consuming that your brain turns off. In the language of psychological trauma, it is as if the brain takes pity on you and injects you with a little mental novocaine to take it down a notch. Our hearts are clenched so hard that they have become stones of despair.

We see Dr. McIntyre near the end of January in his small clinic room on the 9th floor of the VG.

Dr. McIntyre adopts his characteristic listening stance—leaning on a desktop with one arm, while crossing one foot in front of the other. "The pain you are having could result from several things," he says candidly. "It could be nerve damage, radiation damage, or it could be a recurrence of your cancer."

See? That is how you tell patients scary news. Just tell them.

The digital exam is painful. I suppress a whimper.

"You have not used those tissues in a while," he reassures me, "so they are very sensitive. But everything looks good. I do not see or feel anything wrong. Your anastomosis is healing very nicely. But none of this means you are not having a recurrence. So I will order a CT scan to check for recurrence, and a CEA level—a blood test that can be elevated if your cancer is returning. Usually, you must wait until the end of your treatments for those checks, but I will do them now."

"A CT scan would be able to check again for the status of that internal iliac node," I venture.

"Yes, although it did not show up during your surgery," he replies, bending over the desk to complete the paperwork. Inwardly, I marvel at his memory for the insides of so many masked and unconscious people. We are all a set of unique inner roadmaps, and he is the expert cartographer who can recall our different inner landscapes with ease. "But even without that consideration, your tumour was very high risk, so this pain is worrisome."

I leave, the requisition clutched in my hand.

....

The double-contrast abdominal CT scan done by the QEII comes back clear.

I post:

SOME GOOD NEWS
posted by Robin McGee, Tuesday, January 25, 2011, 10:45 AM

Hello RCO:

I just thought I would let you all know the results of my CT scan done last week. No evidence of recurrence, no evidence of metastases, no oversized lymph. It is good news, and in tandem with the low CEA (0.9), indicates that I might be safe for now. Now I just have to stay that way for as long as I can...

I am currently in the second week of a treatment cycle. Each treatment cycle gets a little more difficult. I would say that I am at about 80% energy during off and first weeks. Second weeks, I go down to 60%, and I start to have more pain in the soles of my feet, earlier in the week each time. Fatigue and foot pain seem very trivial compared to the chemo agonies I have heard about from others. Only three more cycles after this one.

DUAL CONSCIOUSNESS
posted by Robin McGee, Thursday, January 27, 2011, 10:45 AM

Hello All:

Many thanks to those who expressed their pleasure at hearing about my clear CT and low CEA levels. I ought to caution people that I am not out of the woods yet by any stretch. To be considered "in remission," one must have no sign of cancer in the body, and to be considered "cured," one must be in remission for 10 consecutive years. My disease was so advanced by the time it was discovered that my chances of recurrences and/or metastasis are rather high—50%—so I don't think I am able to throw a cancer-free party just yet. However, I am glad for any evidence of progress against this killer, so I allow myself some degree of relief.

This 50% thing is very strange. Imagine being told that a Mafioso is out to get you. He has a 50% chance of showing up in the next five years to execute you. And did I mention that he will torture you first? But equally he may not show up at all, and if he does not, you will be safe. Now put that back in your mind and go on with living your life as usual! It is a challenge!

Kris Carr is the young and amazing documentary filmmaker and authour of *Crazy Sexy Cancer Tips*. She describes this dual consciousness of normal life and concurrent dread very well:

"Living with cancer is all about mental management. The creepy thoughts will always slide under the radar. You'll be slicing the Thanksgiving turkey and thinking about how to word your tombstone, watching TV but imagining who your boyfriend will hook up with after you are gone (you may even get mad during this little fantasy, especially if you imagine him with someone younger and prettier than you!). The first few years after my diagnosis, I swear I had an alternate thought track playing on a loop in my mind. Thank God no one asked me what I was thinking about! How I wished I could go back to the carefree innocence that I had taken for granted before the cancer talon popped my little bubble. Unfortunately, there will always be a B.C. (Before Cancer Hijacked my Life) and sadly we can never go back."

This is something I have often wondered about...will I ever be able to live unselfconsciously again? Talking to cancer survivors, the answer is "no"...but they tell me that after many, many years, it is no longer their first and last thought of the day.

Joelle < 1/27/2011 11:35 AM >

Oh Robin, your strength and brilliance and continually inquiring mind always impress and amaze me. I think of you daily, I pray for you daily, I admire you daily.

I know that Agnes always has a cancer loop that runs, even after seven years...and every test that comes out wonky, even a little wonky, sends the loop to the forefront for both of us.

My Dad, who had heart disease since age 45 (and lived to be 79) always said: the trick is to live as if it is your last day and to live as though you will live forever and to do both simultaneously. Know that the warmth of those who love you is near.

Sandi C < 1/27/2011 12:42 PM >

What a good analysis of how your thought processes change once you ever have the diagnosis of cancer. I loved the reference to a Mafiosi threat—what a vivid picture you painted. You are educating us all.

Enjoy your comfort food and keep enlightening us.

Thea B < 1/27/2011 1:43 PM >

I completely understand and can relate to the wish to go back to the Before Cancer carefree, innocent way of living your life. I struggle with that wish as well, not before cancer but before divorce, which is another kind of death and life-changing experience. Yes, it does get easier, and the depressing or frightening thoughts are less likely to be the first thing you think of in the morning or before you fall asleep, but they still rear their ugly heads from time to time. I try to embrace them now, rather than push them away. I think of them as my "character-building friends." By doing that, I am not paralyzed by them as I used to be. When I tried to push them away, they seemed to come back even stronger. Perhaps living knowing that at any time your cancer could return could be a welcomed reminder to live each day with love and appreciation... something that all of us forget to do far too often, and would be so much better off for doing.

I'm buying the tickets for the Mahler concert today.

See you soon and love you lots.

Alison L < 1/27/2011 2:09 PM >

Alison is away this week with her mother on a cruise, but I noticed your email on her computer.

I am sure I can speak for both of us to say we are incredibly pleased for you with your progress. Having a sister who just passed five years of cancer-free, I know it remains an uncertain time ahead. However, this sounds like some of the best news in many months, so we rejoice with you.

The road can be long, but may you celebrate every step of the way.

Very best wishes,

Paul

Susan C < 1/30/2011 5:52 PM >

Good evening Robin,

I know you get many messages, but I just wanted to tell you how much I look forward to your emails. You are a "wizard" with words and I hope some day you consider writing a book and sharing this story of your battle with cancer. It is remarkable that you find the time and energy to do all you are doing, but I am so glad you do. I hope you don't mind that I have started forwarding your emails to my mother and sister. My mom is sixteen years cancer-free and very thankful for every day. My sister has her own health problems with a rather difficult prognosis ahead of her. I think they find your messages inspiring and I wanted to share.

I think of you often and send many positive vibes your way.

Robert McGee < 1/27/2011 6:06 PM >

Having pored over your message, I just have to say that you should be delighted with the excellent results of the CT and CEA. Insofar as the 5-year wait for an "All Clear," just count your blessings. I remember your mother went through this period too, but she always had a positive attitude, and I am sure that helped her beat the beast.

Insofar as 50% statistics are concerned, let me tell you a story. During the war, each Lancaster squadron had 30 aircraft. And one was expected to fly 30 missions. But the squadron lost an average of two aircraft on each mission. So the numbers say that before one could complete a tour, the whole squadron would be wiped out twice over. I suppose one could say that the chances of death/dismemberment were two to one *against* you. But I am living testimony that the statistical approach was bunk. In fact, if one did look at it that way, one would suffer from fear, trembling, and depression. And fear and depression could be fatal.

As you know, I have personally faced death, both medically and physically on a number of occasions. And, at my age, the odds of going on for five years are also against me. But real life ignores odds. I can carry on contentedly, without fear, knowing that there is nothing I can do to surmount the inevitable. Why should I (or you) be worried and unhappy? Let's enjoy life.

Sorry to push unsolicited fatherly advice on you, but I know for sure that you are definitely a survivor. Please know this too.

...with love,

Dad

....

Grimly, Andrew and I drive to our scheduled appointment at the dermatologist's clinic to hear the results of the biopsy. We sit stiffly hunched in our winter coats, waiting for the specialist to come in. We stare at the desk surfaces and papers, trying to slow our breathing. When the dermatologist arrives, he tells us that the pathology results from the biopsy are not available—the hospital lab is backed up. Maybe we could come back in two more weeks to find out the results?

Two weeks later, we find ourselves in the same chairs.

"It is benign," he says. "It was a kind of encapsulated scar tissue. Nothing to worry about."

RELIEF

posted by Robin McGee, Monday, January 31, 2011, 1:45 PM

Hello All:

Today I am writing with relief. Since before Christmas, we have been concerned for Andrew. He had a strange skin growth near his ear, which the doctors opined might be squamous cell carcinoma—the same cancer that Andrew's father died of last summer. We did not blog about this because we did not want to freak out Austin, particularly just as he was going in to exams. We just waited in dread, thinking that having both of us with cancer would be such unimaginable bad luck that we could not process it. We have had to wait weeks for the biopsy results, which were finally available today.

It was benign, praise God. It seemed to be a cyst/scar tissue combination which looked strange and required many stitches, but was harmless. So today we all heave a sigh of relief and go back to status quo.

Austin had his last exam today. We were able to text him with the news before he went in for it. He was, as one might imagine, greatly relieved. Now he has 5 "bros" with him for "bro night," in which he and his friends consume chips and chili and many exploding-helicopter movies. They are outside having a snowball fight right now. Ah, teens!

Joelle C < 1/31/2011 2:52 PM >

Wow, you guys must go off the stress meter…good thing Andrew lives with a great psychologist! :)

Austin's party sounds great...Oh, to be a teen again...on second thought...

Lesley H < 1/31/2011 10:37 PM >

OMG, Robin—I don't know how you managed to hold it together over the last month! I am so glad to hear your good news!

Bless you all—

Jennifer G < 2/1/2011 7:20 AM >

That is such good news! I was reading that note with goosebumps and then tears of joy, thinking about those gangly teen boys romping in your yard like big friendly dogs, including Patrick. How joyful to watch these boys grow up and to see the camaraderie continue from year to year.

Tara S < 2/1/2011 8:21 AM >

Hey!

I can't even imagine what strain you must have been under wondering about this—I'm so glad it was good news!

I'd love to see you—maybe we could get together for dinner or something in the next little while?

28

I AM ON THE LAST CYCLE OF MY CHEMOTHERAPY, AFTER SIX months.

I am weak. As I lie in my recliner by the window, I reflect back on the long winter I have endured. I have not heard any further news from the government, or from the Liberals. When I see him, Dr. Dorreen has continued to provide me with encouraging updates on his efforts to support funding for FOLFOX.

Andrew went back to work two months ago, no longer able to extend his leave to care for me. I have been alone much of the time for many months now.

However, the RCO community have remained persistent in their efforts to support me personally. Some invite me to lunch or activities, some drop by with flowers and gifts, some drive Austin to events. But their greatest means of encouragement has been as the avid audience for my postings.

I cast my mind back to the beginning of winter, and I remember...

THE RESCUE OF DAVE AND OTHER STORIES
posted by Robin McGee, Monday, January 17, 2011, 12:45 PM

Hello RCO:

Today I start chemo cycle number five. Again, side effects are limited to the second week of treatment. I have noticed more fatigue and "hot feet" in the last half of the second week. On the "off" week, I almost feel normal. On the weekend, I went snow-shoeing twice for over an hour each time. It was truly glorious—I think snowshoeing is the reason for winter. I used to be a purist prig about Cross Country skiing, thinking that snowshoeing was for the wuss. I became a convert the first time I tried snowshoeing. It frees one to explore any part of the woods or fields. Truly magic. I may try to get out today if I have time.

Meanwhile, for all you advocates out there—my oncologist told me that the talks over FOLFOX are galloping apace, and that he thinks it will pass the next two committee reviews. If it does, he said, it was because of OUR lobbying efforts. So while it is unlikely that I will get this treatment now, it is very likely to become accepted practice here eventually, which will save lives. Kudos to all of you who wrote the Minister of Health! It just goes to show that social networking can move mountains.

In other news, the Cancer Society has a program that allows one to talk to someone who has survived one's same type of cancer. I talked with a 60-year-old retired teacher the other night, who had a story nearly identical to my own. She had to write the Minister of Health in Alberta to get the colonoscopy that diagnosed her stage III rectal cancer, because her doctor just would not order one despite her year of bleeding!

Also, her oncologist fudged her papers to get her FOLFOX, pre-tending that her rectal cancer was colon cancer. She had trouble tolerating the chemo and had to stop it. She had all the same procedures and surgeries that I will have. It really was helpful to talk to someone who has walked this walk.

One of the things she told me is that after her ileostomy reversal and bowel reconnection surgery, she had to wear diapers for three weeks! Even two years later, she still feels the need to live right next to toilets. Hmmmm...I sure hope I have recovered bowel function before I return to work...but maybe I could drive around in diapers like that crazy astronaut lady! Watch out, schools!

Our other funny story concerns the rescue of Dave, our neighbour's cat. Poor Dave got into our garage woodpile during the terrible snowstorm last week. When Andrew saw him there, cat-phobic Andrew uttered a shriek of terror and surprise. Poor terrified Dave ran up into the garage rafters at this and somehow got stuck there behind some pipes. After several phone calls, we were able to determine that this cat must be Dave, whose family was away in the Dominican. We tried to lure him out with salmon, but no dice. With the enterprise of our other neighbour Nikki Lannon, we were able to get him to nibble the salmon off of a stick. Andrew bravely adorned himself with huge gloves he called "Kitty Mitties," got a transparent box, put the salmon inside it, and murmured endearments. Dave eventually put out his paws, which Andrew quickly wrested, and Dave was free! We slugged through the storm to Dave's house next door, and Nikki, who was housesitting there, confirmed that Dave was very pleased to be home. I have footage of Andrew stroking this cat with his Kitty Mitties, so maybe I have a chance at getting a cat of my own now!

And finally, I heard that Michael Douglas, who has gone through six months of chemotherapy, was very warmly applauded at his appearance at the Golden Globe Awards. He said to the crowd, "There must be an easier way to get a standing ovation."

I will try to post more often and more briefly in the future!

Marilyn C < 1/17/2011 1:39 PM >

No need for brevity on my account—says the woman with whom you spoke for nearly three hours last week! :)

Once I got satiated with answers to my "how's Robin doing?" concerns, I especially enjoyed Andrew's cat desensitization story. Though hardly systematic, it was effective. Should you ever have a problem with a cat in future, call me. I am "the cat whisperer." Actually, my sister-in-law calls me the dog whisperer, but I think my talent there is limited to one golden retriever.

Congratulations on all of your good news! I am holding back on "I told ya so." :-)

Sonya M < 1/17/2011 2:18 PM >

Thanks for the updates and entertainment, Robin! Yee haw about the CEA!! Who the heck calls their cat "Dave?"

Sherrie C < 1/17/2011 7:19 PM >

A good read, Robin. Thanks for the update as we were wondering about you at the soccer facility on Saturday. We are first in the old lady division and third in the young crazy kid division. Enjoying both levels of play. Glad to hear you are out on the snowshoes. Chris, my husband, says it is the best therapy for anything.

Keep up the good work and look forward to the next update!

Cindy H < 1/17/2011 9:00 PM >

There just is not anyone quite like you. I continue to adore you and your courage and sense of humour and steadfast spirit. I want to come and visit you. What is an appropriate day/time for you?

Tell Andrew he has so much courage...I am extremely cat phobic as well!!!!

Hello
posted by Bekki M at Saturday, February 5, 2011, 8:59 AM

Thanks for giving me the link to join your community. I have been reading and following your journey for a couple of weeks now and find myself thinking of you very often through the day. Having a husband who has had aggressive bowel disease for the past 27 years (8 surgeries) gives me a bit of insight into the debilitating pain and some of the symptoms you have to endure. Ron and I are drawn to you and your plight on a daily basis. We are thrilled with each passing tidbit of wonderful news, while remaining realistic about the road ahead. Please know that we send positive thoughts your way each and every day.

SWEET DREAMS
posted by Robin McGee, Thursday, February 3, 2011, 7:45 PM

Hello RCO:

Last night, I had a dream. In my dream, I was visited by two spirits of light, who told me that I would be cured. One was the figure of a man the size of my hand, but indistinguishable of feature and glowing with light. The other, oddly enough, was shaped like a plant holder I once gave my mother in law. It was a square vase made of stone, and on each side was the face of a man. In my dream, this god-vase perched at the foot of my bed, and I sat up to greet it. One of its faces told me that I would be cured, and I thanked it gratefully.

Austin tells me that the idea that angels are cherubs with wings is not founded in the Bible, but rather on Renaissance artwork. The angels described in the Bible are actually very strange-looking— an eye in a triangle with wings, a ring of fire, a towering sound. Maybe my dream visitors were angels? Let's all think so.

Debbie M < 2/3/2011 7:57 PM >

That is very beautiful. Sounds like angels to me! You must feel immeasurably comforted.

Lesley H < 2/4/2011 2:07 PM >

Wow! What a beautiful visitation!

I believe they were angels.

Bask in the light and hope, Robin.

Grace M < 2/3/2011 8:05 PM >

I believe in angels. I hope that these were angels and that they were forecasting the truth! This dream and Andrew's medical news makes this a very special week! I am sending you huge, huge hugs!!

Take care!

Suzy and John < 2/4/2011 11:20 AM >

Let's hope that Austin is right because those little plump putti that show up everywhere in Italian Renaissance art are ador-able—especially attractive to developmental psychologists like we are—and surely they should be your harbinger of good news. Let's also hope that spring is coming and bringing a relief from cold along with good health.

Stefani H < 2/4/2011 9:24 AM >

The dream you blogged about was beautiful and inspiring Robin. :)

And a plant holder is intended as a vessel to contain a living, growing thing that contributes to the cycle of life and wellness for our planet—hmmmm...

By February, advocating members of the RCO community had started to receive the email that Minister MacDonald had sent to me.

MAUREEN MACDONALD'S EMAILS
posted by Robin McGee, Friday, February 4, 2011 8:36 AM

Hello RCO:

All those of you who lobbied Minister MacDonald are now receiv-ing a FO and D email from her. She is just getting around to responding to all of you, having sent me the identical email before Christmas.

She says that no one has brought FOLFOX forward to the Cancer Systemic Therapy Policy Committee as yet. Actually, that is changing as of this month! A group of oncologists at the QEII, inspired and emboldened by our lobbying, is preparing a brief for this committee as I write. My oncologist, who is head of the department at the QEII, said the forward motion on this initiative is directly attributable to me, to us, to all who emailed the Minister. He seemed so grateful, even relieved, to have a reason to argue for this treatment, knowing as he does that it is so much more aggressive than what they can offer now. A friend with the same cancer, from Alberta, told me her oncologist faked her papers in order to get her FOLFOX! All the experts know this is the right treatment for patients with lymph involvement. Thanks to all of you, that treatment could be available to cancer patients next year.

In all likelihood, it will be too late for me to receive it by the time they ratify it. I have only nine more weeks of treatment to go. My last day of chemo will be 3 April.

I will keep you all abreast of how the FOLFOX fight is progressing. We have set such a great and good example of how social networking technology can change society. Someone should do a thesis!

CHEMO CYCLE SIX
posted by Robin McGee, Monday, February 7, 2011, 9:45 AM

Hello RCO:

Today I started cycle number six of eight. I am finding that each cycle gets a little harder. I am at about 80% energy during my off week, but it drops to 50% in the second treatment week. But I hope to have enough energy today to attempt snowshoeing out the back yard, as it is so beautiful here today.

Today I am wading through my income tax. As part of that enterprise, I must input all my income from my private practice.

In reviewing the receipts, I find myself very moved by seeing the names of my former private practice patients.

My private psychology practice was very tiny—only three patients a week. However, I had done it for over 15 years, so I saw many, many people there. Mostly adults, although I saw the occasional child or youth.

As most of you know, I truly love my day job as the Consultant for Psychology Services at the AVRSB. However, my private practice was the setting where I could practice psychotherapy, which is a great love of my life. Last year, I had some tremendous treatment successes, which were immeasurably rewarding and inspiring. I had several patients who were not just restored to minimal function, but who emerged from therapy literally glowing with mental health. Much of that is due to a wonderful therapy protocol for trauma that I have learned, Eye Movement Desensitization Reprocessing (EMDR) therapy. I recall one session with a woman who had been savagely raped by a stalker. She raised her wondering eyes to mine after she had finished her protocol and said, "I have been living with rape trauma for 20 years—and now it is gone. GONE!!" Her happiness in her work, life, and family became joyfully evident in subsequent sessions.

As news of my illness spread through the Valley, many past patients wrote or called me. One wrote: "There have been many therapists in my life, many of whom helped me a lot. But it was with you that I felt really changed. You have such a keen balance of insight, listening, and playful banter that created the safe space for me to deal with stuff I had been working through a long time." Feedback like that has been a great solace and inspiration to wellness for me.

It is a strange feeling to be on the receiving end of a patient's concern. However, it is a frank and compassionate encounter when both therapist and patient are humbled by fate and the human condition. I like to think that when I am well again, I will be even better at psychotherapy. Sometimes, the depth of one's

ROBIN MCGEE

personal suffering, transmuted by the discipline of psychology training, can make one wiser and more empathic.

God willing, someday I will return to my private practice. I can't wait.

I remember times when my courage failed me. Behind my house are fields that go on for miles—in winter, a white expanse broken only by the occasional stand of trees. Before I became too sick, I was able to snowshoe there.

One afternoon, I ventured into the whiteness alone. I went further, beyond the borders of my usual foray, and kept going. Blue shadows over the white drifts drew me on, as in a dream.

All at once I realized that I had gone beyond my strength. I no longer recognized where I was; everything was white, nothing could be distinguished. Suddenly, I became afraid that I might not make it back. It was like an apt metaphor for my cancer journey.

I sank to my knees, unable to continue. The wisps of snow that ran over the surface of the endless white swirled around me. I heard the rasp of my own breathing and the piccolo of the wind. Nothing else.

The smartphone in my pocket chirruped. I fumbled it out of my parka and read:

Marla D < 2/7/2011 11:24 AM >

Dear Robin,

I religiously read your notes and am so humbled by your intellect, compassion, and courage. As long as I have known you, you have challenged and inspired me. You continue to do this as you battle cancer.

I just wanted you to know that in addition to the changes you help your clients to make, you make a positive difference to me too.

Keep up the good work!!!!!

After reading that message, I was able to struggle to my feet. I could keep going, and find my way home.

FOOT PAIN BLUES
posted by Robin McGee, Monday, February 14, 2011, 9:00 AM

Hello RCO:

I am heading into week two of chemo cycle number six. Two more cycles still to go. The side effects get worse with each cycle. I now have more fatigue as well as the beginnings of "hand and foot syndrome"—in which one's hands and feet become extremely hot and sensitive. In bad cases, the soles of the feet and the palms of the hand will blister and split. I am not at that place yet. But I am experiencing some difficulty walking, as the soles of my feet are "sunburned." I used to experience that on day 13 of my cycles, but now I have it on day 7. So with each cycle, the "bad" aspects creep forward, happening earlier each round.

I have to slather my feet with udder cream, keep them elevated, put ice bags on them...you really don't appreciate the soles of your feet until they are compromised! Curiously, my hands are red but not sore. Still these sufferings are nothing at all compared to what my father-in-law went through with his chemotherapy, so I continue to feel grateful that things are not worse.

While slathering my feet today, it struck me forcefully that I will never play soccer again. This is a realization I knew in my mind, but somehow it hit me emotionally today. My team captain has asked for my shirts back, but I wonder if she should retire my number—after all, my number was unlucky "13." Maybe I can learn to feel better about this loss when I find some substitute physical activity. But I miss soccer and all my teammates, more than I can say.

Maria C < 2/14/2011 11:04 AM >

Robin, we miss you too!! And we still do a cheer for you at the end of each game (win or lose). Although you may not play with the team again, you are still a Raven and can join us at any time. I think of you often and faithfully read your updates, and I am so pleased that while the feet may be sore, there are more upsides to your situation at this time.

Heather M < 2/17/2011 11:40 AM >

Keep your feet up, Girl! These treatments won't last forever. We miss you every single game and I cannot wait until the Blomidon dinner so we can "hang." Dig deep and let all that stick-to-it-iveness you've got on the field pull you through this battle off the field. Hey, maybe our little soccer team was just a kind of basic training for you...

Shirley E < 2/17/2011 12:30 PM >

I can totally empathize with you about the treatment symptoms multiplying as time goes on. I found the last three rounds quite hard and I'm not sure if it is mentally or physically. I seem to be grinding to my feet instead of jumping. My fingers were all wrinkled up this time and when I touch my bald head, my feet get a zinging sensation. So far, I haven't had peeling feet but they are very dry; their scratching on the sheets drives me crazy. It's bound to happen but at the same time I am grateful like you.

My QiGong teacher told me to chant:

> My blood and qi (chi) are flowing smoothly and beautifully
> I am filled with peace and joy
> I am free from pain and illness
> I am blessed with good fortune

I do this while I am working around the kitchen or driving or wake up in the middle of the night. It is telling the brain what to believe and know so it can send the right messages to the body. I believe in this mantra. You probably have your own.

I will be thinking about you in your next few treatments and cheering you on. I find out the results of my CT Scan tomorrow. I'm hoping to be clear or at least have some reduction so I know we are going in the right direction. Have you tried acupuncture for your symptoms? I always feel much stronger after those sessions.

Sorry about the soccer but why can't you play again?

I reflect on the ways I have found to cope with the pain of my temporary ileostomy. Over the months, I have consulted regularly with my Enterostomal Therapy Nurse Eleanore Howard. Fifteen years ago, Eleanore and I had both served on the same small Child and Youth Mental Health Team at the local hospital. She left the team to become a specialist in stoma and wound care, and in a fortunate turn of fate, I am now her patient. Eleanore has taught me ways to care for my excoriated skin: using powders, using hairdryers, using patience. She tells me that permanent end ostomies are more stable and easier to manage than temporary loop ones like mine. She researches different appliances that push down the skin around the stoma, giving it a reprieve from the acidic stool that seeps from underneath the seal. The new appliances helped at first, but we have learned that the deeper more convex appliances have given me pressure ulcers around the stoma. Eleanore listens supportively to my angst. I am touched by her tenderness and responsiveness to me. I cannot imagine confronting the problems of this ostomy without her, and I wonder how people do it who do not have access to enterostomal therapy nurses.

Andrew found a website that sold one-size-fits-all tube tops, and I bought several. These garments hold the appliance more firmly in place and allow me more secure freedom of movement. I have learned how to become more active with it. However, as I become increasingly compromised by my chemotherapy, my activity level is falling away.

The RCO blog has over 200 members. I knew that someone on the RCO blog might someday end up with an ostomy. I hoped to normalize the experience.

I posted:

LIFE WITH FLIPPER
posted by Robin McGee, Monday, February 21, 2011, 12:15 PM

Hello RCO:

Several of you have asked what life is like with an ileostomy. We call mine "Flipper" because of the strange dolphin-like sounds it occasionally makes. My Flipper is a projection of my small intestine, so he allows me to digest while I am "disconnected" from my large intestine. He allows the large intestine to heal after surgery.

I both hate and love Flipper. I love him because he spares me from the worst tortures of chemotherapy—diarrhea and constipation— which many chemo patients will tell you were both their agony and their danger throughout their treatment. If I had ulcerative colitis or Crohn's disease, I would definitely consider a Flipper because he gives total freedom regarding travel and food choices.

I hate Flipper because he is a lot of work. Dealing with him is gross, but no more gross than dealing with a baby or a dog. My Flipper is very small. He is surrounded by a plastic skin barrier, and his head is covered with a cloth pouch. Like some kind of strange prairie rodent, he raises his little head above the skin barrier, looks around, and then retreats back under. When he is under the barrier, he can burn me with the stomach acids he works with. Consequently, the skin next to him is often badly scalded. To try to keep up with him, I have to change the skin barrier seal every other day. Thank God for my private insurance, for those seals are 10 bucks each!

I will get to say goodbye to Flipper in May, praise God. He gets tucked back inside me. This will be a half-hour surgery, not a 5.5-hour surgery like I had in September. But then the real suffering starts. After nearly nine months of not being used, the large intestine has to figure out how to function again. By report, this is a very arduous process. Survivors say they had to wear diapers for weeks. However, I know both Flipper and I will be happy to have him home where he belongs, no matter what the cost.

The other day a friend suggested we go to a spa to get "pampered." I said this sounded like a good idea, because soon I will be wearing them!

Debbie M < 2/21/2011 12:28 PM >

I see a David Cronenburg film in this...

Judy K < 2/21/2011 12:23 PM >

Oh Robin, God love your sense of humour.

Grace M < 2/21/2011 1:30 PM >

Thank you for describing your ileostomy—so many people never want to talk about it. I appreciate your sense of humour. You certainly see the glass "half full."

I love the name—Flipper. I wish that we had thought of using a fun name like that when my Dad had an ostomy—Great idea!

I think back to the supportive care I sought over the winter. The horror of confronting the four percent had shaken me so much that I knew I needed psychological help. When I told an oncology nurse at the Cancer Centre about my distress, she responded that the wait for therapy through the psychosocial oncology team there was at least two months. Unless I had a comorbid condition like bipolar disorder, I would not be seen in a timely way. She urged me to find a private therapist, a task that I managed alone.

I had several sessions with counselor Mary Goodman, of EastWind Health Associates. Warm, thoughtful, and supportive, she listened actively to my anguish. I spent many sessions simply crying, trying to wipe away the tears of grief over leaving my family bereaved or sentencing them to the agony of watching me die slowly. Alternatively angry and anguished, I voiced to her my sense of hurt, betrayal, and frustration with Doctors One through Four for putting me in this place. Throughout, Mary was my respectful witness. She taught mindfulness practices that helped me to stay in the present and stay myself.

Too sick and too distant from the various in-person support groups, I knew that nighttime winter travel was out of the question. Lloyd, the leader of my local Canadian Cancer Society support group, kept me informed by email of online webinars and opportunities for care.

I remained so internally injured. The dilator is a miserable, unlovely experience. Andrew jokingly refers to it as "the Dildo of Damocles," as even looking at it evokes such fear and dread in us. We are two frightened people who cling to each other each night. The expressions of tenderness that would naturally melt into intimacy are now thwarted by pain. An aspect of our marriage that had always been so fun and healthy is now complicated and sad. *Will I always be this damaged?* Only Andrew's patience and sense of humour keeps me grounded. I know I need guidance.

I learned through the Cancer Society about an opportunity for such help. The award-winning nurses Dr. Deborah MacLeod and Joan Hamilton offered an online chat group on women's sexual health. Using the online support platform Cancer Chat Canada[2], the technology allowed me and several other cancer survivors to "chat" by typing. Each week for eight weeks, I logged into that receptive community. It was safe, both physically and emotionally, to go there—a fact I often reflected on as I listened to the winter wind scream outside my house. All the other participants were breast cancer survivors. One had had both breast and ovarian cancer—18 years previous! I was the only participant in active treatment. The group had been reassuring, hope-giving, informative, and fun. Andrew and I often joked about "the sexy nurses" who advised us

2   www.cancerchatcanada.ca

about how to cope with my complex of radiation and chemotherapy symptoms.

One day, when I was in the Cancer Centre, I was approached by a friendly woman with curly hair. Her eyes were magnified by thick glasses that did not conceal the glint of humour there. She asked me if I was Robin McGee, and when I affirmed my identity, she said she recognized me from my chatroom avatar. Nurse Joan Hamilton and I shook our hands; from that day forward, she has become my champion, advisor, and ally. She has met with me, shared books with me, sought my opinion on resources, and ran interference for me throughout the health system over various medical difficulties.

I think of Joan gratefully as I lie weakly in my chair by the window. She had won the CCNS Excellence in Patient Care Award the previous year. To me, she is the personification of the word "medical excellence."

HOPE

posted by Robin McGee, Friday, February 25, 2011, 9:30 AM

Hello RCO:

I saw the oncologist again yesterday. A resident came out to greet me. She shook my hand and gazed into my face, saying, "It is an honour to meet you! Dr. Dorreen has told me what you have done to help oncology!" When Dr. Dorreen joined us, he said that the application to extend FOLFOX to rectal cancer passed through all the internal hospital committees. It will go before the provincial Cancer Systemic Therapy Policy Committee next month. "It is a shoe-in to pass," he said. He thanked me again for adding a new weapon to his arsenal against cancer. I told him to call me as soon as it is ratified, so I can send word to all of you. Thanks to this community, the Minister of Health received nearly 100 letters advocating for this change.

My bloodwork was good, so I do not have to go back until June! They thought my feet were good enough to proceed on the same dosage of chemo for my last two cycles.

I am posting under "Resources" the article I recently published in the Association of Psychologists of Nova Scotia newsletter. It is a brief piece describing the emotional and ethical struggles I experienced when closing my private practice. I have had lots of heartwarming feedback on it from psychologists across the province.

My son Austin is the sound geek for the "Women of Wolfville" production going on this week. He seems to be loving it, and he is certainly learning how complex theatre sound work can be. We went to see it last night. The theme is "Hope"—something I could use these days. Something that seems to be growing for me.

When my paper entitled "How to tell your patients you have cancer: A psychologist's journey" is published in our provincial association newsletter, several of my colleagues reach out supportively.

David P < 2/23/2011 8:34 PM >

Dear Robin:

The Nova Scotia Psychologist arrived in the mail today and as I flipped through the contents, I came across your article. I read it right away. I want to thank you for writing such a moving, brave, and thoughtful piece and for sharing your story in such a public way. You humanized an unthinkable situation and you offered a very relevant professional perspective on something that many of us would not know how to respond to. Psychology is blessed to have you as a part of our community. Thank you!

I do hope that your health continues to improve and that things are going as well as when I saw you last in December. I trust that your family is doing well also.

Lauren M < 2/24/2011 8:53 PM >

Hi Robin,

It was wonderful to chat (and eat) with you a few weeks ago. You are a Psychologist's Psychologist whom we all personally and professionally admire and I was so impressed to hear you were sharing your journey with others. I would be honoured to have access to your blog if you are comfortable with that. I'll be yet one more person sending you all the energy I have and anything else you need.

Over the course of the winter, it dawned on me just how much of a financial drain this cancer has been and will continue to be. I encourage others to buy into critical illness insurance that can protect them from such devastation.

EXPENSIVE!!!!
posted by Robin McGee, Tuesday, March 1, 2011, 1:15 PM

Hello RCO:

I have started cycle number seven of eight. There is a light at the end of the chemo tunnel! By report, the last two cycles are the toughest in terms of side effects and fatigue. My feet and hands will likely start roasting next week. Right now, they are wrinkled and dry but not actively sore. Last week, when I was strong enough in my "off" week, I resumed working on my taxes. This time, I was tabulating medical expenses. No one ever tells you how *expensive* cancer is! In 2010, my 44 drives to the hospital came to nearly $5,000 in mileage alone. My lost income, even with Long Term Disability support, will be approximately $100,000—more if I cannot start work in the fall. None of this includes the cost of the drugs, supplements, supplies, and parking. Those add up to many thousands more.

Shirley E < 3/1/2011 10:22 PM >

Hi Robin,

Interesting that you should write about the cost of cancer as I was doing up my medical stuff for income taxes. We are so lucky in New Brunswick (NBTA) that we are 80% covered under our Johnson plan for almost everything, with no age limit. Our union bargained long and hard for the benefits under a group plan. My sisters in Nova Scotia, who were also teachers like me, are looking at the same plan you are talking about. I'd hate to think what my cancer has cost in total, but the amount spent for drugs alone just this year was $39,000. This does not include the chemos given at the hospital. My cost was $8000, which was taken up mostly by the Victory Program. Some patients die here because they have no insurance plan that covers the extra drugs and, in my case, the unusual ones. My trips to Sweden cost in the realm of $5000 for the tests and consultation each visit, which my plan covers if Medicare doesn't. I pay for the flight, food, and hotels while there.

I would also advise anyone to buy into a plan. Hope you have an easy two more rounds. I know the mental fatigue sets in as well as physical about now. But you are almost there!!!! My thoughts are with you!!! SD

Andrew's return to work has been challenging for him. To keep his job and his benefits while caring for me and coping with his own incapacitation, he had been metering out a career's worth of accumulated sick days by taking as many hours without pay each week as he could. However, his sick days were running out, and we know that he will need some left to help me after my reversal surgery. So he has gone back to work as a senior project manager for a large engineering consulting firm.

I can see how difficult the transition has been on him. His company has merged with another and his office has been moved since he has been on cancer duty. His responsibilities typically demand a high level of concentration and dedication over the course of long complex projects. While he stayed home to look after me, his longtime understudy had assumed his role as the leader of a specialized machine design team. So when Andrew returned to work, he was offered a new and unfamiliar role available due to the sudden departure of a manager from another team. Now Andrew has to provide leadership to a team he has never met before and who specialize in a field of engineering for which he has no background. There is a lot to learn, and the shock is telling on him. He has spent the past year living day-to-day, afraid to think or plan or hope beyond the next few months. Now, he is forced to think and plan for an entire work team, all the time not knowing if this is the end of my cancer odyssey or just the opening chapter.

We both worried about how I would weather the days without him. He has been my number-one caregiver, supporter, and confidante throughout so much. But we have no choice. Although I am often lonely without him at home, I reflect that his return to work restores some aspect of normalcy to our shattered lives.

I am saddened to think about Austin. My cancer has thrown Austin off the dock—it is all he can do to tread water. Sensitive to but overwhelmed by my illness, he tries valiantly to cope by denying his own needs. He tells us repeatedly that he is "fine" and that he "does not want to burden us." Increasingly, he declines to attend the social events he used to enjoy. He does not discuss his stressful situation even with his closest friends, and he rebuffs our offers of counseling. Despite his stoicism, we see the toll it is taking on him. His schoolwork and marks suffer as he gradually withdraws into the escape of music and the internet. Some teachers are supportive, emailing me about his missed assignments and the drift they see in him. Others are not, and give him no quarter. I often reflect that any working adult in his situation would be granted a stress leave, but students are expected to continue on without reprieve. When I think of the damage done to my child by my avoidable situation, I am filled with impotent rage against Doctors One through Four. But my sorrow and anger on Austin's behalf are mingled with my own shame: I have become too weak to sustain normal domestic responsibilities, and he increasingly assumes them. I take his avowals of wellbeing at face value, too sick to do otherwise.

ATLANTIC PATH

posted by Robin McGee, Wednesday, March 23, 2011, 9:30 AM

Once more into the breach!!!

It is day three of chemo cycle eight, my final cycle. I am looking forward to this cycle ending, while having some dread about it: final cycles are usually the harshest.

What does this chemotherapy feel like? For me, it feels like a combination of being clubbed over the head and being burnt from the inside out, miserably spiced with dehydration. When the feet get problematic, the sensation is just like walking over a hot beach—ouch, ouch, ouch!—with every ginger step. Right now, I feel like a desiccated stick insect. The palms of my hands are shriveled like those of a 90-year-old. Nevertheless, all this is still much better than my poor father-in-law went through, with his head in the toilet for months on end. (He was treated before the good anti-nausea drugs were available). Only two more weeks, and I can begin my recovery.

I do not yet have a date for my surgery. I am praying for end of April beginning of March. I really want to have it done by my very esteemed surgeon, who retires in June. I have told his secretary that I intend to stalk him if he retires beforehand. I plan to hide in the bushes by his golf course, and sprint out and prostrate myself over the putting green, holding aloft a scalpel!

Have you heard about Atlantic Path? Nova Scotia has the highest rate of all cancers than any other province, and researchers are trying to find out why. This is a huge study, planning to recruit thousands of participants and follow them over 30 years to figure out the determinants of cancer. I have volunteered to help recruit subjects by appealing to the RCO community. I myself have enrolled (you can still participate even if you have had cancer). Andrew's entire workplace has enrolled. What is involved? You must complete three questionnaires about lifestyle and family history and send in body measurements and toenail clippings.

(They are looking for arsenic in your toenails, thought to be high in NS drinking water). For those of you in Ontario, a similar study is underway. I have posted the study recruitment info under "Resources" on the website.

Colleen R < 3/23/2011 10:39 AM >

Hi Robin!

So glad you are on your last cycle—I will pray for it to go smoothly for you.

I wanted to let you know that I already signed up and sent in questionnaires for the Atlantic Path research, back around Christmas time. Another friend of mine is a recruiter.

It's wonderful you are so proactive for yourself and others who might follow in your path. You are an amazing human being.

Caroline W < 4/11/2011 12:21 AM >

Please forward my contact info on for the Atlantic Path research.

Glad that the chemo is finally done and you have a date for surgery.

When out in my garden today, I thought of the bulbs we planted last fall. Hopefully they are poking up through the soil and will be in bloom soon for you to enjoy.

Thinking of you often.

Grace M < 3/23/2011 4:13 PM >

Good luck with this final round of chemo!

I participated in Atlantic Path study last year. Went to Halifax and completed the assessment—painless, but very worthwhile!

CRAWLING TO THE FINISH LINE

posted by Robin McGee, Saturday, April 2, 2011, 10:15 AM

Hello All:

I am now crawling to the finish line…only two more days of chemo-therapy and this Olympic event is over. I have withstood this last cycle reasonably well, but I have had the foresight to do virtually nothing, as any activity is draining and hard on the feet.

I am launching an appeal for yard help! I need to rake my lawn, and I am not allowed to wear gloves or even stand for very long. Maybe I will be better in a few weeks. I have put an appeal on the calendar for Sunday April 17th.

I have a surgery date! It is now set for FRIDAY THE 13th of May(!). Maybe 13 is a good number for me. It was my soccer team jersey number. In my books, any day is a good day, as long as my superlative surgeon does the procedure before he retires. Looks like I won't have to stalk him after all.

The other day someone told me that his dog was promptly scoped after rectal bleeding. It is both miserable and ironic to realize that a dog can get better medical attention than I could. But Andrew had a witty quip for that one: perhaps if I had been "their collie, instead of their colleague," the doctors in my case might have paid attention!

I just booked a weekend for Andrew and I to spend at Trout Point Lodge at the beginning of May, the weekend before surgery. Expensive, but the food is said to be great, and God knows when I will be able to eat decent food after the surgery. I want to sit in on the deck in the sun. Let's all sing along with George Harrison and the Beatles: Sun, Sun, Sun, here it comes.

Allison M < 4/2/2011 5:11 PM >

Hi Robin,

It's Allison here. I've been following your journey and trying to do my little part from away. I guess I'm living proof of the butterfly effect. Your battle has really brought perspective to my life and has also ingrained some important lessons...nothing to the extent of what you're currently experiencing, but I have already switched doctors because of the dismissive (and I'd go as far as saying sexist) attitude I was given. I suspect your story has affected people from one end of the country to another, possibly further.

Anyway, I am interested in participating in the Atlantic Path study. I have forwarded the information to many of my friends and family. I was surprised to find out my mother volunteered last year!

Judy K < 4/2/2011 6:15 PM >

You are indeed a remarkable lady. You have fought this fight with dignity, laughter, and head-on determination. We are all praying that the outlook is good and we will have you back with us soon. It is hard working without your guidance to back me up—I depend on you...

...so God, you have to be listening and make Robin all better for herself, her family, and all of us.

Sonya M < 4/3/2011 10:49 AM >

Thanks for the update and I'm so happy that you have just about made it to the finish line without too much distress. I won't be signing up for yard work for two reasons if I am to be completely honest: 1) I'll be in Florida and 2) even if I wasn't, I hate yard work! OMG about the dog!!!! I think you'll love Trout Point. Ian and I were there last year at the same time. It is fabulous.

Linda G < 4/4/2011 9:51 AM >

Good to hear you are indeed reaching the finish line of this race…
and so happy to hear the surgery will be following quickly and by
someone you trust. He has you in good hands! And from all He's
done to use this medical crisis of yours for the benefit of others,
it is most impressive. And glad to hear you and Andrew haven't
lost your sense of humour! Hope the trip away gives you time to
reconnect and reflect on life after this is all behind you!!!

Love you. You are all in my thoughts and in my prayers…

Patricia B < 4/2/2011 8:31 PM >

Dearest Darling Robin,

As always, your bravery and stoicism astonish me…

I hope you have at least been able to read and watch movies. Is
your appetite still good or are you having nausea? I've got your
surgery date marked on my calendar so I can send especially
powerful thoughts your way that day. I think that a weekend away
before your surgery is a great and romantic idea. In the long
run, I bet you'll have wonderful memories and the cost will be a
non-issue.

I'm hoping you are energized by the coming of spring after this
beast of a winter—the days getting longer, the little spring flowers
poking up, sighting of the first Robin! (You see, you are a harbinger of spring for me). I really wish I could volunteer to come and
rake your lawn…

So much more to talk about—let's have phone call soon.

Love you deeply.

Pam S < 4/4/2011 8:35 AM >

Congrats on this being the last of the last and getting a surgery date!! I miss seeing you—so could you sign me up for the Atlantic Path thing??

The 13th is such a lucky date—it will be another in the series of Robin wonders—I know!

Here comes the sun dootin doo doo

XXOO

....

My reflection brings me to the present. Here I am, chairbound.

Xeloda's side effects have caught up with me. The fatigue is grinding. All my mucosae have dried up: the inside of my nose, mouth, and throat have become parched. The "hand-and-foot syndrome" has left the underside of my hands and feet hot and raw. Now, the skin is coming off my soles in sheets. It is painful to walk, and I can no longer hold utensils. Bloodwork from the Cancer Centre shows my red count and my lymphocytes to be very low. When Austin comes home after school, he finds me unable to stand. He cooks the meals and does the dishes before starting on his own homework.

I spend my days in my chair by the window, my feet elevated. Austin is busy around me: cooking, cleaning, offering me tea.

Once I was a busy mother who managed an active household. Now, my child looks after me. Once I was a hardworking clinician who used to regularly cross the province and even the continent in pursuit of my career. Now, I am lucky to even cross my own living room. Once I was an active athletic person who worked out regularly—I could play three games of 7-Aside soccer in a row. Now, I cannot even stand up. Every identity, every outward manifestation of my self, has been stripped away.

But I still have options. I can open myself to feel the love and kindness of others, the support of good and decent clinicians, and the tenderness of family.

Austin comes in the room with my tea. As he gives it to me, he hands me a letter.

It is from the College of Physicians and Surgeons of Nova Scotia.

29

THE COLLEGE HAS DECIDED TO DISMISS MY COMPLAINT against Dr. Number One. In their opinion, her misdiagnosis of my symptoms as due to an antibiotic reaction was a reasonable decision; after all, I had been on antibiotics when the symptoms started. They considered her ignorance regarding C. *Difficile* test standards to be understandable, as she had no experience with these requirements.

I am disappointed that the Committee did not address the *omissions* of Dr. One, such as her failure to order bloodwork, take into account my family history of colorectal cancer, arrange follow up, or refer me for endoscopy. I check the envelope: there is nothing about Doctors Two, Three, or Four. *They must have something stronger to say about them*, I hope.

Another letter arrives a few days later. Investigation Committee B would like to interview me on May 15th.

I call them to say that I cannot make that date—I will be in hospital only days after my reversal surgery. The assistant I speak to is not impressed. She suggests that I will have to be interviewed by telephone. When I say that the matter is too important to do by telephone, she replies that they do not have another committee meeting scheduled for months—telephone is my only choice. I tell her that I will not cancel my surgery, but that I would do anything else in my power to meet with the committee in person.

She calls back a few days later. The Chair of Committee B will be in Halifax on other business and is willing to meet with me on a different date. No, I cannot meet with the whole committee: only the Chair and the public representative will meet with me. Patients are rarely invited to talk to the investigation committee, but she tells me that they sometimes consider it "in serious cases." Because my documentation was so thorough, meeting with me is really only a formality. I am allowed to bring a support person. When I ask if the doctors will be allowed to meet with the full committee, she replies that she is not at liberty to disclose that information.

So they consider mine a serious case.

Andrew and I arrive at the CPSNS offices. It is only a few days before my reversal surgery. We are ushered into a small waiting room.

My heart is pounding. *Please God make them listen.* My anxiety comes in waves: *I am responsible for protecting the lives of other citizens. I have to get this right.* If I am not clear enough, if I am not persuasive enough, then other Nova Scotians could end up as I did. My suffering and my possible death would be in vain, as no doctor would be any wiser and no patient would be any safer. But with each heartbeat of anxiety comes a counterwash of clarity: *the College itself is responsible.* The individuals on the investigation committee have the true burden of public protection. I can only tell my truth to power. I cannot make them *hear* me.

After a half hour, we are brought into the big boardroom. The Committee Chair greets me respectfully as "Dr. McGee."

He introduces me to the woman serving as the public representative. She regards me with serious eyes in a drawn face. The rest of the people in the room are clerical staff.

After we are seated, the Chair invites me to share anything else I want to add, above and beyond my written submissions. The woman joins with him in thanking me for the thorough and complete way I had documented the case, making their job easier.

I have a few prepared notes. For each of Doctors Two, Three, and Four, I try to convey to them the flavour of each encounter with each doctor. As I speak, the emotion evoked is so powerful that

Andrew must sometimes place his hand gently upon my shoulder to settle and support me.

I ask them to look at my face, and see that mine is the face of the public they are meant to protect. I ask them not to be misled by my appearance: all four of the doctors in my case had dismissed me because I was "not pale." I point out that Dr. McIntyre had described me as "remarkably well-looking" when he simultaneously documented that I had a tumour the size of a grapefruit. I read from documents that underscore my grim prognosis.

"I deserved from those doctors," I say, "appropriate assessment for serious symptoms. As all patients deserve, regardless of our faces. Besides," I add, "if we could tell who had cancer and who did not by looking at them, we would not need doctors!"

One of the clerical staff stifles an ironic laugh.

"I was an educated middle-class articulate allied health professional. I was even on a first-name basis with two of these doctors. If care this bad could happen to me," I challenge, "what the *hell* is happening to the woman from the trailer park?"

They listen attentively and inscrutably with few questions.

The Chair respectfully holds out my coat for me.

We are led out of the room by one of the clerical staff. "If there is anything I have learned from working here for years," she confides to us, "it is 'never get sick.'"

"You were the perfect balance," Andrew says in the car afterwards, "of eloquence and restrained emotion." He could not imagine me doing a better job. I know it to be true: after all my careful documentation and impassioned appeal, if I cannot make CPSNS hear me, then nothing and no one ever could.

It takes weeks for the decisions to arrive by mail.

There are four levels of discipline that can be meted by the College of Physicians and Surgeons.

Dismissal of the complaint can occur where there is insufficient evidence that the care provided was below the acceptable standard.

A Counsel is a warning given when a doctor's care may have fallen below standard and where he or she might benefit from guidance.

A Caution is given when it is clear that a physician's conduct has definitely fallen below standards. A Caution "is an expression of the Investigation Committee's dissatisfaction with a physician's conduct or care and to forewarn the physician that should the actions reoccur, more serious disciplinary action may be considered...the Committee considers a Caution to be a notice of a serious nature."

A Reprimand is the fourth level, typically reserved for criminal levels of conduct or very serious impairment. Reprimands are expensive, as they can result in costly hearings.

For anyone in a regulated profession, a Counsel or a Caution means somewhat more than those words imply. They represent significant humiliation: a body of one's peers has witnessed and judged your failure, and has put you on record for it. Doctors with consciences would be deeply ashamed of a Caution or even a Counsel. However, only reprimands are made available to the public.

Doctor Two received a written Caution. The letter says, "the Committee is of the opinion that Dr. Two failed to include pertinent information in the referral letter to Dr. Four, such as your family history of colon cancer and the results of the rectal examination. The referral letter did not include the risk factors for significant bowel pathology which would have described the clinical picture of your presentation and the reasons for the request." They added: "The Committee considered this to be important information that may have assisted Dr. Four with the triaging of the complaint and may have facilitated you in receiving a colonoscopy in a timelier manner. It may also have been helpful for Dr. Four to have been made aware in the consult letter that Dr. Two was leaving her practice and what her plan was in transferring your care, to help ensure follow-up." The letter added in italics: "*Investigation Committee B therefore issued a written Caution to Dr. Two of the importance of including all pertinent clinical information in consult letters to assist the receiving physician with the triaging of consults. And, furthermore, to inform the receiving physician when leaving or closing her practice, to assist with follow up and transfer of care.*"

Doctor Three also received a written Caution. The letter explained that he apologised to them for his many failures. He provided them with a number of changes in his office process he implemented since receiving the complaint. The Committee was in agreement that the actions that Dr. Three did not do should have been completed. They "found it disappointing that Dr. Three did not follow up on his offer to inquire about the status of your referral for a colonoscopy and that this appeared to have been overlooked in his office, as well as your subsequent call of July 2009 to his office." The Committee was "also of the opinion that it would have been prudent for Dr. Three to have conducted a physical examination with a rectal exam, and not to have relied completely on a previous examination conducted by another physician...Although the Committee was reassured by the changes he has made to his practice and office procedures since the complaint, it was of the opinion that serious discipline was warranted based on the number of concerns it has identified, and Dr. Three has acknowledged, as aspects of the care that should have been conducted in a more prudent manner." In italics, my letter added: "*Investigation Committee B therefore issued a written Caution to Dr. Three to be diligent when assessing patients, by including his own examinations when appropriate, and to be diligent as a patient advocate, by ensuring that appropriate follow-up occurs through his conduct and by having the necessary office procedures in place.*"

Dr. Four, the general surgeon, also received a written Caution. When she was interviewed by the Committee, she reported that she had a "new process" for triaging referrals for acuity and for communication of expected wait times to referring physicians. She reported that she now met with her office staff on a regular basis to review pending consults so that triage was no longer left up to her receptionist. However, the Committee was "disappointed that practices Dr. Four now has in place were not present when your referral was sent to her office. It may have been beneficial for you to have been able to speak to Dr. Four or be accurately informed of the expected wait time and of other options that may have been available to you." They were disturbed by the inaccuracy of both her previous triage approach and the inaccuracy of the information her office had given me. They wrote: "because of its concerns regarding the organization and delivery of Dr. Four's care in 2008, the Committee is of the opinion that a Caution is warranted." In italics, they added: "*Investigation Committee B therefore issued a written Caution to Dr. Four to personally and actively maintain an accurate triaging system for consults and to communicate with family physicians and/or patients accurate information regarding expected wait times.*"

It feels so strange to be holding these letters. Although the fact that the doctors were disciplined is vindicating, a Caution seems so inadequate. I remind myself that I knew—had known from the first—that no higher punishment could occur. After all, their actions were not criminal. In my view, the Committee did not address some of my fundamental objections to the terrible care I had received, particularly the failure of all four doctors to warn me that my symptoms could mean cancer. But then again, the Committee had detected errors of care that I did not raise, such as Dr. Three's failure to examine me and Dr. Two's failure to communicate that she was closing her practice. So maybe it balances out some way in the end.

Perhaps uncharitably, I am glad that these doctors had been made to squirm in front of an investigating panel of their peers. I am certain that the process caused them anxiety. But I also know that no matter what nervousness they each underwent as they sat in that glass-walled office, their sufferings could never *ever* compete with mine.

I am disturbed that there seems to be no real mechanism to ensure that the doctors will follow the explicit directions they had been given. I would have liked Dr. Four to undergo a practice audit to find out what had happened to the other patients waiting 15 months for consultation, like me.

Out of respect for the College process and the privacy of the doctors in question, I never post on the RCO blog about the College complaint. Only a handful of my closest friends know about it.

Although it is difficult for lay people to believe, the truth is that there is no connection whatever between a College discipline and medical malpractice law. College decisions are not even admissible in a malpractice action. Likewise, Colleges never learn of nor act on malpractice suit outcomes. Doctors who have been successfully sued many times continue working with impunity, with no one the wiser. Just as with vehicle insurance, they do not pay one personal cent towards the damages they inflict—it is all covered by their malpractice insurance. The government heavily subsidizes the Canadian Medical Protective Association (CMPA), which provides malpractice insurance and legal defense for most doctors. Those who are successfully sued do not even pay higher insurance premiums, as the payouts are absorbed by the entire medical profession, and the premium increases that result are spread out among the profession as a whole.

The two venues have different objectives. The College wants to ensure that expensively trained doctors are up to minimum snuff. Therefore, the doctor's assurance or other evidence that they have "changed" is sufficient for the College. In contrast, a court of law does not care if a doctor pleads he has reformed. If I run over your child with my car, it will not avail me in court if I protest that I have since taken improving driving lessons. In a court, the concern is whether there is a generally accepted standard of medical care that the responsible doctor failed to meet and whether this breach caused harm to the patient. If these criteria are established during litigation, the CMPA may compensate the patient for the resulting damages. Cancer patients with little time left must often choose between a College action and a malpractice suit. To provide for their families, many go with the lawsuit. Most people, sick, injured, damaged, or dying, do neither. However, the public should be aware that *only the College* has the power to compel change in a doctor's practice. The law does not.

It is estimated that over 100,000 Canadians die from medical malpractice each year in Canada. Those are the deaths, not the injuries. If a fatality rate that high were found in the airline industry or even the military, Canadians would be up in arms. As the damaged and dying usually have other things on their minds, the true number of complaints is greatly underreported. But the system that regulates doctors relies on the College complaint "witchhunt" system, which ignores the role of systemic factors. A better system would mirror the process employed by the airline industry: when dangerous mistakes are detected, all aspects of the system are reviewed.

In my heart, I ponder whether I can ever forgive those doctors. Technically, for true forgiveness to occur, the offender must realize that they have done something wrong—they must be sorry. I try to imagine those doctors as they began their careers in medicine: as idealistic, hopeful, eager to help others. None of them had gone to medical school to neglect cancer patients to death, and none of them had actively intended to kill me. However, their evasions and prevarications through the College process were disheartening. How can I forgive them if they do not take responsibility, if they are not sorry? It seems to me that my forgiveness would mean nothing to them. For Dr. Four, in particular, my forgiveness would be as meaningless as to an unblinking lizard.

Many a time as a therapist, I have sat across from people who have been damaged by human agency. I have seen people savaged by criminals, damaged by reckless drivers, scarred by pedophiles. I know very well that much of human suffering is caused by the malice or negligence of others. In some of these cases, it can help the victim to think that they were simply unlucky, that they were in the wrong place at the wrong time. But who would ever think that going to the doctor when you are in trouble is the wrong place at the wrong time? Besides, I like to think we can hold our doctors to a higher standard of conduct than those of drunk drivers or serial killers.

Where does all this leave me? Only in the same place where too many have been before me: damaged by others who do not want forgiveness, who see no need for it. When the criminal defrauds you of your life savings, when the sexual predator takes your child's innocence, when the politician poisons your water supply—can these acts be forgiven? How ought we to respond when those who require our forgiveness do not even recognize it? Forgiveness can be waved away by those who disdain it. What can you do if your agonized effort at forgiveness is yawned at, or openly scorned? Or if they blink at you, uncomprehending?

You can meet your undeserved fate with resolve. You do not have to forgive, but you can accept. You can see your victimizer for who they really are. You can surrender to the fact that some people cannot change. They are too broken, too defensive, too incapable of insight. After all, with some perpetrators, you cannot make a silk purse out of a sow's ear. When the ideal of repentance is unattainable, we must still come to closure, even if just in our hearts.

Dr. Three attempted an apology, feeble as it was. Of the four doctors, he was the only one who voiced any regret or remorse. Below the patina of hurt, beyond the awareness of grievance, lives my memory of his best self. Despite all his many failings as a physician, I know that he is a human being of conscience—someone who is ashamed to have seriously neglected a trusting patient. For that reason, I see him as somehow greater than the other three doctors; sometimes, I can imagine extending my forgiveness to him, because he once sought it.

When technical forgiveness is impossible—when the one who hurt you is dead, defensive, or indifferent—closure is still possible. You can surrender your resentment and cynicism in order to remain openhearted to all others. Acceptance is the altar. On it, you lay who they are and who you are. You can set the altar ablaze and watch as your past is consumed by the conflagration, offering the story to a watching Heaven. Or you can turn and walk away from the place of sacrifice, leaving it exposed but untouched. There is a dignity in either choice. Acceptance is the gift of peace that you give to yourself.

I wonder if anyone will be safer because of my complaint to the College of Physicians and Surgeons. *I did my best,* I whisper to the world, *under very trying circumstances.*

30

I AM SHIVERING IN MY JOHNNY SHIRT IN THE ANTEROOM TO Dr. McIntyre's sigmoid clinic. The strange pain I have in my phantom rectum has persisted. In a few minutes, Dr. McIntyre will check me for a possible recurrence. The words of his last report race around my disordered mind. "Her pain is worrisome," he had written, "given her previous pathology."

My heart is pounding so hard that I can see the front of my Johnny shirt jumping. *This is fear of recurrence,* I recognize. Desperate, I review every self-soothing trick in my psychology arsenal. I try each of them, one after another: deep breathing, emptying the thoughts, mindfully noticing. I fiercely remind myself that I have already been through so many challenging and brutal procedures that I can get through this one thing. I swallow a bolus of fear. But my heart still pounds.

Dr. McIntyre is flanked by his usual entourage of medical students and a practice nurse. After a few preliminaries, he beckons me to mount the examination table.

After he puts in the scope, his next words are cheerful.

"Everything looks good. The scar is healing so well you can barely see it." He turns to the students, "Come over and see this! If you look here, you will see the anastomosis scar and a little staple." I hear and sense the students crowding around my upraised bum. Through my dizzying relief and embarrassment, I note with amusement the note of enthusiasm in Dr. McIntyre's teaching voice:

"...and if you look here, you can see the colon!" *After 31 years*, I think, *he still can get excited about teaching this stuff.*

When I am back in the patient chair, my reprieve is translating to a relief so dizzying and intense that it is difficult to form questions.

"If you are still having that pain," he was saying, "we should consider taking another image."

"I have had three CTs in the past 10 months," I say. "Can we do an MRI instead?"

"That makes sense," he replies. "I want to know you are clear before I operate again. We also need to double-check about that right internal iliac node that was seen on your diagnostic imaging. Ostomy reversals are usually superficial. We just sew the stoma shut and poke it back in. It takes about a half hour. But I can go in where I first cut you and take a look around—maybe do more if we have to."

I shudder at the thought of my surgery scar reopened.

"I need to remind you," he continues, "just because your images are clear does not mean that you are not having a recurrence. Sometimes they take months or years to grow to where we can see them and deal with them."

I nod. Living with the threat of cancer is like being a mountain climber. Just as you scale a blind peak, you see another treacherous vista and another precipitous drop before you.

....

Dr. McIntyre's secretary Leslie Snide confirms a tentative surgery date. Ever supportive, she calls to affirm that she has sent the requisition for a preoperative MRI.

The date for surgery is getting closer. Even as I fear the inevitable dysfunction, I long to be free of Flipper. But I have not heard about the MRI. I grow uneasy: something is wrong.

I call the imaging department at the QEII. I learn that the request for the MRI was redirected to my local regional hospital. You have to call them, not us, they tell me. After several fruitless calls, the mystery is solved. The fax machine at the imaging department of

Valley Regional Hospital had run out of ink, so all faxes received that day were ignored.

The MRI has to be re-ordered. Because he cannot risk not having the results in time, Dr. McIntrye is forced to postpone my surgery.

CATCH-22
posted by Robin McGee, Wednesday, May 11, 2011, 3:45 PM

Hello RCO:

The surgery has been rescheduled to the 24th, but still may need to be cancelled again if the Radiology Department at the local hospital does not get the information to the surgeon on time. Yesterday, the local MRI unit told me that they typically require two weeks. They shrugged off the problem that the surgeon needs the findings within eight working days—"he can look at it himself," they said, "or he can get a radiologist from his own DHA system to look at it." So health districts simply do not cooperate or coordinate with each other, and the domino effect of this affects individuals, families, inpatient units, workplaces, etc. My surgeon's secretary promised me she would call them every day to get them to provide the results as soon as possible. Let's hope that the radiologist does not "dig in" and stall out of spite, as the staff there have previously hinted that urgent requests are put at the bottom of the pile on purpose because one of the doctors does not like being told what to do. I feel like I am living in a Joseph Heller *Catch-22* novel, in which everything is the opposite, and you cannot win for losing.

Very soon I shall post my spiritual musings as a result of this journey. Having cancer is not simply walking through the valley of the shadow of death. At my stage, you have to move into that valley, break out your dishes, and put up the curtains. You have to fill your bookshelf. I have done that, and done a lot of reading and wondering. More later.

When I first started this journey, I talked with other cancer patients. Each one warned me about this stage: chemo is over, and you are awaiting the first set of scan results to see if treatment worked. They each told me that undergoing that first CT, MRI, or mammogram is fraught with apprehension. I recall one woman telling me that her legs gave out on the steps of the building as she tried to march to her first post-treatment mammogram. At the time, I remember thinking that I would be so lucky to even make it to this phase, so I hoped that I would not be unnerved when the time came. It is not entirely rational to be so trepidatious; after all, it is what it is, and taking the photo does not change it but only reveals it. Nevertheless, this part of the journey is particularly and humanly challenging.

When my MRI is finally scheduled, I go to my local hospital. I recognize with gratitude that the technician who comes to assist me is the same woman who had so graciously helped me during my MRI the year before. Her compassion for us, knowing of Ron's imminent death, resulted in her expediting my imaging, arranging a CT on the same day as that MRI. I share with her how grateful we all were to her, because her thoughtfulness meant we could say goodbye to our loved one.

She shrugs modestly. "You had the IV in anyway," she says. "It only made clinical sense...it seemed like the efficient thing to do."

As I am slid into the MRI machine, I give thanks for the small mercies of attentive and human health care.

....

With only weeks before my reversal surgery, I know that I need more supportive care. *I must prepare myself for whatever that MRI will find,* I tell myself. *I must accept it.* I have gratefully joined an online webinar on mindfulness. Radiation Oncologist Dr. Rob Rutledge and Counsellor Dr. Timothy Walker wrote *The Healing Circle*, a book of remarkable cancer biographies about real people. I had read it shortly after my own diagnosis. In addition to the astonishing stories of courage and acceptance, the book contained guidance regarding coping techniques such as mindfulness meditation, yoga, and movement practices such as Qigong. The online webinar was the leaders' first attempt to reach people using such technology; usually, they presented information in weekend workshops.

Each week, I pull up to my computer to watch the two of them. Although the technology frequently bogs down, their sincerity still shines through. They lead exercises in yoga and meditation. Most importantly, for me, they introduce via live video some of the survivors profiled in *The Healing Circle*. Many of these patients had experiences and pathologies as harrowing as my own. Each week, I am greatly heartened to actually *see* those survivors, as their faces swim up on my computer screen. The book had been published the year before and the manuscript was older than that, so all these people had survived very grim situations. *They are still alive.* Seeing them gave me hope that some people can survive even against extraordinary odds. And Dr. Rutledge and Dr. Walker are reflective and respectful, sharing their message of mind-body healing with grace and warmth.

Concurrently, I read books on mindfulness meditation. I try it for weeks, devoting at least 20 minutes each day to it. As I do, I notice its impact at other times of the day: I see the greenness of grass, hear the hum of birdwings by the window, taste the tang of spaghetti sauce.

I post:

SPIRITUAL MUSINGS
posted by Robin McGee, Friday, May 13, 2011, 1:15 PM

Hi All:

The MRI was yesterday. I was surprisingly calm throughout, even falling asleep in the machine. The techs had to wake me up. It was like being in a warm cocoon for 30 minutes. I feel relieved to have made it through that experience. And now comes the wait for results, which any cancer patient will tell you is one of the worst steps on the journey to endure.

I have promised to blog about the spiritual side of this challenge. So many of you have asked. By saying what I will, I do not wish to disparage anyone's religious tradition or beliefs, only to describe my own searchings and thought processes.

No one can confront cancer without some kind of spiritual awakening. I have read accounts of atheists facing their prolonged cancer deaths; I have great respect for their bravery and perceptivity as they surrender their lives. Most of them seem to focus on and take comfort from the fact that nature goes on without them, and to reflect on the good deeds or contributions they made during their lives.

I am not an atheist. I have, at times, tried to adopt an atheist perspective, but it always fails me. I can't help it: I am a believer and always will be. It is something I just know, in my bones.

If pressed to identify my religion, I would say that I am a Christian. Not only is this my culture and my ethnicity, but it reflects my irresistible attraction to the character, example, and courage of Jesus Christ. The only God I could respect is one that entered into our sufferings. Jesus knew, as I do now, what it is to dread a terrible death. Jesus knew, as I do now, what it is to be betrayed by those you thought you could trust. Jesus knew, as I do, how hard it is to speak out against what is wrong, and how sad it is to see the sufferings of others. I lose patience with those New-agers who say that Jesus was so blissed-out on God Consciousness that he felt no pain on the cross. I love Jesus mainly *because* he underwent so much pain. The pain I share with the suffering baby in the hospital, the shuffling little old lady, the anguished who struggle with mental illness, with all other cancer patients, and with all of you.

I have been reading extensively in other religious traditions recently. In particular, I have read several books by Buddhists: Pema Chodron, Chogyam Trungpa, the Ripoches, and Vietnamese monk Thich Nhat Hanh. These writers emphasize mindful acceptance and celebration of life in each moment. I have found their ideas to be very soothing and wondrous. Thich Nhat Hanh suggests little concrete techniques to experience life's joys: for example, when you hug someone, you should hold the hug for the space of three mindful breaths to stay present with the loved one in that hug. Try it! These writers as well as non-religious psychologists advocate for mindfulness meditation as a means of acquiring peace. Although my Western mind cannot always follow the metaphors of Buddhism, I try to grasp the main principles, which ultimately lead to responding to the world with loving kindness.

Also, I have been reading a lot in the tradition of Judaism. In particular, I have been reading books by Rabbi Harold Kushner, who wrote the famous *When Bad Things Happen to Good People.* With his knowledge of Hebrew and his understanding of the great Rabbis of the past, he interprets various scriptures and ideas. Of all the theologies, I find his to be the most sensible and compelling. He summarizes it in six words: "God is moral, Nature is not." Nature is blind, uncaring, and incapable of distinguishing among us: nature does not make exceptions for nice people. The natural world has much beauty and is lawful in its underpinnings. However, it does not have the attribute that we have—the ability to judge the difference between what is morally right and morally wrong. Our responsibility, in this theology, is to bring as much knowledge, beauty, and active compassion as we can into this world. And God gives us the strength and comfort to do so.

I do not see cancer as a gift. I would never give it to you for your birthday ("Oh Robin you shouldn't have...just what I was missing...a carcinoma"). Life is the gift: cancer is what makes you more aware of that.

....

It is the day after my MRI. I am pulling up dandelions in my back yard. I work stolidly. When my fear about the scan results threatens to become unbounded, I breathe. I see the ground, feel my muscles pulling, feel the heft of the garden tools in my hand. *Mindful acceptance*, I pray. *Acceptance.*

My son Austin comes running out of the house with the tele-phone in his hand. "It is Dr. Good!" He cries. "It is for you!"

I take the receiver into my hand and hold it to my ear. All the world goes still.

"I have your MRI results available. They just came in," says Dr. Good's gentle voice. "It is clear."

The sun, the grass, the trees—everything flies away like a cloud of starlings.

"Let me read this to you," Adam continues. "It says 'No pelvic lymphadenopathy is seen. There is one small right internal iliac node with measures 0.5 cm short axis. This node is at a similar location as the previously seen mildly enlarged node which had measured 1.2 cm'...and the summary impression says, 'No pelvic adenopathy by size criteria. Apparently, no nodes were removed at the time of surgery. This suggests that potentially the previously seen right internal iliac node was enlarged on a reactive basis and has since returned to normal size'...Robin, this means you should be free to go ahead with your reversal without issue."

Austin is anxiously searching my face. I repeat aloud what I hear Dr. Good say. Austin sways and falls back a few paces.

When I punch the phone off and lower it, Austin rushes into my arms.

"The angels!" he crows. "The angels in your dream said you would be cured!"

I laugh. "But you don't believe in angels."

"I do today," he shouts, swinging me around.

With our arms still around each other, we go back inside the house and collapse on the couch before our fireplace. We take turns playing our favourite celebration songs on the BOSE. When Andrew comes home, he finds us head-nodding together.

I post:

CLEAR

posted by Robin McGee, Tuesday, May 17, 2011, 11:15 AM

Hello RCO:

The results from the MRI have come in and they are...CLEAR! The wonderful Dr. Adam Good phoned me at home to tell me. My first MRI one year ago suggested I had a distant lymph node involved. If that node was cancerous, I would technically be stage IV and hence incurable. Worse, this node's involvement is so lethal that I would only have a 4% chance of survival.

That node did not show up on the two CT scans I have had since surgery. And the MRI shows this node as back to normal size. So it was either reactive, the way lymph nodes can get, and not cancerous in the first place. Or it was an artifact of the first MRI image. Or it was involved, but was down-staged by the radiation treatment. Whatever the explanation, these results confirm that I have a 50% survival chance, not a 4% chance.

This means that I can go ahead with my relatively superficial surgery next Tuesday...Flipper begone!

And the Community responds with joy and congratulations. Within 24 hours, over 55 people in the RCO community personally email to express their heartfelt relief.

Thom W < 5/17/2011 1:19 PM >

Hi,

It has been bleak and rainy here for days and days, and we had a flood last week. Suddenly, everything feels so, so, so much better.

Tears to my eyes!

Margie N < 5/17/2011 12:25 PM >

Robin I am so thrilled for you to get this re-affirming news, especially as you head into your surgery. I hope it makes everything you have ahead of you that much more manageable, although by no means pleasant. I had the thought as I read your message that even though your experience with doctors has been so awful, Dr. Good is a star that shines as an example of what we all want... medical *care*, not just medical treatment. I am so thankful you found him and I am so thankful, from a selfish place, that he is taking such good care of my friend!!

Lisa P < 5/17/2011 12:22 PM >

That is the best news, Robin!! What a huge relief. Remember that that 50% is based on the general population too, so it's likely your chance is sooooo much higher given everything you are doing for your health, your mental attitude toward this, and all of the emotional support you have from friends and family.

Rob B < 5/17/2011 12:09 PM >

Fabulous news, just fabulous!

Roger and Joan < 5/17/2011 1:41 PM >

Dear Robin

I am delighted! Thank you for letting us know about your clear test.

We'll be praying every day, but especially on Tuesday—that the 50% will change to 100%. Whatever the explanation may be, God is good. And Adam Good is mighty good too!

Marilyn C < 5/17/2011 3:22 PM >

...And of course, while perfectly lovely to hear, this news does not surprise me at all!!! :)

Sheila M < 5/17/2011 11:37 AM >

Wonderful news!! It no longer seems like an overcast day!!!!!!!!!!!!!!!!!!!!!!!

Cheers!

Joanne P < 5/17/2011 7:29 PM >

Dancing with joy and tears in my eyes. I love you. Take care.

Lady J

Darlene W < 5/17/2011 9:39 PM >

YAHOOOOOOO! Reading your emails, I never know what to say and usually don't respond, but I am so glad to hear that you heard good news that I couldn't resist.

Neives L < 5/23/2011 5:14 PM >

HIGH FIVE ROBIN!!!!!

WOW! I am so happy to hear this.

I read it fast when you sent it, but didn't have a chance to let you know how excited I am for you!

Now you can repeat to yourself as a mantra: THANK YOU, I AM FREE FROM TUMOURS. THANK YOU.

I will certainly send you thoughts of light and healing tomorrow at 12 my time.

I am sure everything will be all right.

Lots of love.

Joan B < 5/19/2011 3:45 PM >

I am overwhelmed to hear your news—all the way to us in Morocco! You have survived an incredible trial and been a wonderful witness to us all. God bless you.

Heather M < 5/19/2011 5:59 PM >

So ...does this mean you are coming back to the team this summer or do we have to wait until next summer to bring lucky number 13 back to the field? I am overjoyed Robin! What miraculous news! The sun IS shining! FINALLY!

Best of luck ridding your life of the useful, necessary, but unwanted Flipper. Remember him fondly. I'm sure little Flipper was a journey of his own.

Love, Heather

P.S.

Yay!

31

OVER SEVERAL MONTHS, I HAVE DEVELOPED THE IDEA THAT I ought to nominate Dr. McIntyre for some kind of award. Cancer Care Nova Scotia has an Excellence in Patient Care Award. Established in 2008, the awards were intended for those clinicians and groups that contributed the most to cancer care. The process requires the nominator to complete the nomination forms, write a letter of nomination, and acquire at least two other letters from others. I have work to do.

When I share my plan with Leslie Snide, his secretary, I ask her to keep it secret from Dr. McIntyre, at least until after my reversal surgery. She sends me his curriculum vitae, from which I start to build my case. I email a request for a letter from a fellow patient, a university professor whom I know indirectly. His eloquent reply arrives the next day. I am touched to see from the date/time stamp that he must have composed it during the wee hours of the morning. I also acquire a letter signed by three of the province's enterostomal therapy nurses. I take a day to compose the strongest nomination letter I can.

As a result of Dr. McIntyre's retirement, Leslie has to find a new job. I have written a heartfelt letter of recommendation for her. I reflect that after all the secretarial ineptitude I had encountered with Doctors One to Four, Leslie has taught me that medical reception can be safe, sensible, and supportive.

There is one more surgery to get through in May. I should learn the results of my nomination when the CCNS Awards are declared in June.

I post:

FAREWELL TO FLIPPER
posted by Robin McGee, Sunday, May 22, 2011, 8:45 PM

Hello RCO:

Well, I had my last meal. Andrew and I went to the Port Pub to load up on the sustenance I will need to make it through the next two days of no food at all. Only liquids tomorrow and nothing on Tuesday, surgery day. After going nearly six weeks on a liquid diet this time last year, going two days will be a breeze.

I must be at the VG for 10 am on Tuesday, with surgery to take place three hours later. Send me your positive vibes!

I am so looking forward to my fond farewell to Flipper. Necessary and hardworking Flipper will take a final bow, and all the organs and cells in my body will give him rapturous applause. He certainly "took one for the team." Afterwards, I will think of him warmly, nestled as he will be among his fellow intestines, resting after his yeoman's service to me. And all my internal organs will welcome him home as the hero he is.

....

I am in the preparation room for the operating theatre. I find it hard to subdue my enthusiasm. Because Dr. McIntyre has two surgeries before mine, I have come prepared to wait. They tell me he is running behind. The nurse that prepares me for the OR tells me again how lucky I am to have him as my surgeon, and how much they admire him and will miss him once he is retired. "He is the very best there is," she says simply.

When I am finally wheeled into the OR, it is nearly 5:30 pm. As the staff prepare me, they look at the consent form I had signed earlier in the day.

"You have written here that you want Dr. McIntyre to do the procedure." They look at each other ominously and one even groans aloud.

"Yes," I say, not understanding. "I do not want a resident to do it."

I push the play button on my ipod. My guided imagery mp3 for successful surgery swells in my earbuds, and I go under.

I awake in a dark hospital room in the VG. Three other patients are sleeping quietly. Andrew stands above me.

"It's late," Andrew says. "Past 10 o'clock. There were complications. Dr. McIntyre found some scar tissue was holding your stoma in place, so he had to open you up through your original incision. It took a lot longer than planned."

My hand steals under my blanket to my stomach. Underneath the gauze I can feel the ridge of staples going up my abdomen. But when I move my hand to the right, I feel another patch of gauze where the ostomy had been. I fill with elation. Flipper is gone.

The next few days are a miasma of unconsciousness. I have fleeting recall of nurses bending over my bed to take my vitals. The pain is far less than the first surgery.

I look up to see Dr. McIntyre at the foot of my bed.

"You came within an ace of having your surgery cancelled," he says. "That morning, I had two very difficult surgeries before you. The first one was the worst case of Crohn's disease I had seen in 25 years. But that was only until the afternoon, because the *next* person I saw was truly the worst case of Crohn's disease I ever worked on. You were supposed to be a quick pop-it-back-in, but it became clear in a few minutes that was not going to work. I was going to have to go in through the original incision and do the takedown from underneath. So I removed the scar tissue and adhesions that were causing the problem. That scar tissue was what caused your emergency obstruction last fall."

So that obstruction was never my fault, I think, softening.

"...and while I was in there," he continues matter-of-factly, "I took some extra time to take a look at that iliac node everyone was worried about. I had a good look at that lateral chain area. It was fine, just like last time."

My drug-addled mind wonders vaguely if Dr. McIntyre will part his white coat to display the Superman symbol beneath. After he leaves, it dawns on me slowly why the OR crew had groaned aloud when they read my consent form specifying that Dr. McIntyre was to do my procedure. They were empathizing with the exhaustion he must have felt after two arduous and complex surgeries. I sink back into my bed, my astonishment transforming to awe.

I hug to myself the secret of his nomination. I wonder when he would be notified of it, and if he will be pleased to hear of it.

But just before I leave the hospital, an email arrives from the Award Committee at CCNS. The message says Dr. McIntyre has not won the excellence award. Instead, it has been given to truly impossible competition: a group of nurses who volunteer their summer vacations to run a camp for children with cancer.

I call Leslie, his secretary, to schedule my post-op consult with him. She books it for the end of June, only a few days before his retirement.

"He got the letter of nomination," she confides. "He was tickled to get it. He still does not know who nominated him." Together, we hatch the plan that I would give him all the nomination materials at my final meeting with him, so that he could at least see the salutary letters and comments made by his colleagues and patients.

I leave the Victoria General Hospital. It feels so astonishingly freeing to walk out of that building for the last time, and without an ostomy. I watch the spring sunshine on the Halifax buildings, see the lovers strolling on the grass. I am going home.

HOME FROM THE VG AT LAST

posted by Robin McGee, Saturday, June 4, 2011, 2:30 PM

Greetings to Everyone:

Well, I am finally out of the Victoria General and back at home sweet home. Man, it is good to be back.

What can I say about hospitalization? It was easier to endure than the first two times, probably because I knew what to expect. But it was still very harrowing. Those of you who have seen floor 9 of the VG know that it is like a World War I field hospital: wounds everywhere, screaming, no room to move, harried nurses running from bed to bed. There is no air conditioning there, and the rooms become stiflingly hot. One nurse told me that last August the temperature in my room went up to 55 degrees—even the staff were vomiting. There certainly is a need to tear that place down and build a new hospital, as that one is ancient.

On a few nights, I had very intense pain, likely due to mistimed liquids. I felt as if someone had attached a bicycle pump to my insides and pumped until all my internal organs were at the screaming point. The same thing happened to two other people in my room—one an 80-year-old woman who ended up with an NG tube. It seems that the dietary food-delivery people did not properly respond to the doctors' orders about our fluid restrictions. And another night, the poor demented man in the bed across from me tore out all his tubes, vomited on himself and shat himself, and screamed helplessly for his mother for hours. In the close, hot room, the stench was overpowering and nauseating. The nurses let me sleep on the couch in the solarium because there was no other bed. That was the toughest night.

But some aspects of my care were excellent and astonishing. My surgery was delayed by many hours because, ahead of me, my valiant surgeon operated on two people whom he later described as the two worst cases of Crohn's disease he had seen in 25 years. Both were unexpectedly complex, and he had been operating since 7 am. Despite all that, he refused to allow my surgery to be cancelled, and I went in to the OR at 5 pm that same day. Expecting me to be a straightforward, half-hour procedure, he discovered that Flipper was refusing to go back in due to an adhesion. So he had to reopen my original incision and fetch Flipper from underneath after removing the scar tissue. (He also said that this adhesion was the reason for my emergency bowel obstruction last fall). So a half-hour surgery turned into a two-hour surgery for him, after a very grueling day. And despite all that, he was still absolutely thorough, careful, and meticulous. He even went beyond the call of duty to look around for any problem or malignancy when he was inside, just to be extra certain I was clear—over and above my MRI results. So although I have experienced the very nadir of medical care, I can also say that I have experienced the very pinnacle of it, in the professional and conscientious person of my heroic surgeon, Dr. Bernie McIntyre.

And in the middle of the night early after my surgery, the nurse at my bedside was taking my vitals and readying my injections. She noticed a little silver angel I had on my table, a slender gift passed on down through four other cancer survivors to me. When I explained to her the story of this angel, and told her that I was to pass it on in turn, she smiled. After she had administered my treatments, she reached up to gently caress my cheek. A little gesture, but it meant a lot to me.

And now I am home. We are all so exhausted. I am sleeping much better now that I do not have to tend to Flipper. Bowel function is, well, a puzzlement. I was warned to expect uncontrolled diarrhea for weeks, but what I seem to experience the most is the opposite problem. I no longer have a rectum, so I have no muscles to help with the process; so things are very slow-going, as it were. Think of rabbit pellets (and then don't think about that!). My skin is quite sore and sensitive. I have been to the drug store to buy all the products I have not used since Austin was a baby: Zincofax, Tucks, baby wipes, etc. I am staying very close to home in case of accidents, but I am hoping that gradually things will become more predictable. *Sigh*. My previous experiences have taught me to be patient, so I will be patient.

Coming home, I also realize that I will need help soon with various tasks. I will need another "garden help" day. I am wondering about next Sunday, June 12. I need help weeding and planting some annuals. And now that summer seems to be approaching AT LAST, I need help exchanging the winter clothes for my summer clothes in my closet. The clothes are all too heavy for me to lift.

Thanks again for all your prayers and good wishes—I am grateful for every single one.

32

I AM IN THE CANCER CLINIC FOR MY FINAL MEETING WITH Dr. Dorreen. I have been out of hospital for two days.

He is pleased with how I have done overall. Relatively speaking, Xeloda monotherapy had been easy for me. He explains the path for future follow up: CEA levels taken every three months and a CT scan once a year for three years.

"And I have something else to tell you," he says with a grin. He sets down his papers, folds his arms on the table, and leans toward me.

"This is a Pyrrhic Victory for you," he says, "but a victory nevertheless. FOLFOX is now approved for use with node-positive patients with rectal cancer. The Deputy Minister of Health and Wellness for the Province of Nova Scotia signed his formal approval on the 31st of May—last Friday. I have two patients starting on it this week."

That was the day I left hospital, I realize.

He sits back, obviously chuffed. "We should have done it years ago, but as you know there was never the Level One studies to support it. We have you to thank. If it had not been for you, none of this would have happened."

"I passed you the ball," I say, "but it was you who put it in the back of the net." I smile inwardly at my soccer analogy, which means more to British people.

"At the last minute, at the last committee, the government baulked," he says. "They did not want to pay for it. But by then it was too late—there was just too much support, too many things that had happened."

Dr. Dorreen gathers his papers and stands up. "The next time I meet you, Robin," he says warmly, "I hope it is socially."

He extends his hand and I grasp it gratefully.

When he leaves, Andrew and I cross the room to each other and embrace silently. Nurses and doctors walk past the open door. The conversation and noise of the clinic is all around us. We stand there wordlessly, our arms around each other.

The chemotherapy event is over.

··········

I post:

WE DID IT!!!!!!
posted by Robin McGee, Tuesday, June 7, 2011, 8:30 AM

Hello RCO!

I saw my oncologist the other day, hopefully for the last time. He told me that only a few days ago, the province finally approved FOLFOX for node-positive rectal cancer. He has some patients starting on it this week!!!!!

He was mightily pleased, saying this change should have happened years ago. The situation needed, well, us. Our lobbying made the difference. He said at the last minute the government hesitated, saying the treatments were too costly. But by then the groundswell of support among oncologists and pharmacists and others was too powerful, and the government finally consented.

YOU should take a moment to congratulate yourself and this Lotsa Helping Hands online community. We have changed the face of cancer treatment in this province, through our collective voice.

I still struggle to recuperate. Still hoping for some garden help volunteers this coming Sunday. I hear the sun will shine...

Eventually, the CCNS website reveals the approval process through the Cancer Systemic Therapy Policy Committee. The record therein shows the history: it shows Dr. Dorreen's background documentation, the projected costs and benefits, and the formal recommendation. The vote and recommendation to fund had taken place in March.

The gratifying word stands in bold capitals beneath my blinking cursor: *Approved*.

So much struggle was represented in the achievement of that word. So much personal integrity lay behind it from so many players—notably Dr. Dorreen and Diana Whalen. Behind the scenes, the Minister of Health had responded honourably as well. It is rumoured that even Premier Darrel Dexter had taken an interest in seeing this through.

All of it had come about by a miracle of mutual readiness: public pressure, research findings, restless oncology, conscientious civil servants, and responsive politicians. All those elements had combined like music to bring about such fundamental change.

Still, for me, there is an element of bittersweet to this outcome. I had victoriously crusaded for that therapy, but was denied its benefits. Like Moses, I could lead other patients to this promised land, but I could not enter in myself. I smile when I consider those patients who would undergo the challenges of FOLFOX. I am sure they would laugh derisively at it being considered "the promised land." But some of them will enter into the promised land of full recovery because of that treatment. My own story is unfinished, and my own survival uncertain. I know that I may yet die a martyr to my own cause.

But when the RCO community learn of our accomplishment, they respond with joy and jubilation at our victory.

Colleen R < 6/7/2011 4:12 PM >

Hi Robin,

I'm not entirely sure why I have these tears in my eyes right now. Although to know I may have played a small part in such a big movement has something to do with it. To know that there are people who may LIVE because of your initiative must be amazing, Robin. Without your hard work, insight, and laying it out there for us (it was so easy just to send an email), it would NOT have happened. What an amazing legacy for you!!!!!

I send you and your family warm and loving thoughts. Remember all those Robins you talked about? Are they all still around? Perhaps you can give the fears to one of them to hold on to, and she can take them into a back room only to come out when you invite her. She must be a strong one—one who will be loyal at all costs to you, the Robin who wants to go about her day-to-day activities with joy.

It is amazing to think of all you have gone through and are going through. You have always been a wonderful person, Robin, but the number of lives you have affected in a positive way has exploded through all of this. Through your suffering, SO MANY PEOPLE have benefited. Me included, as your heartfelt messages remind me to cherish every moment of health.

Thank You.

Lesley H < 6/9/2011 7:17 PM >

YEAH! I am happy to hear your news, both about how you have changed the system for the better for all Nova Scotians (you deserve an award!) and about your bloodwork. Hearing your honest and brave stories all the way along continues to challenge, educate, and open me. Thank you so much for this precious gift, Robin. Although I hope I never have to experience what you are going through, I will undoubtedly have my own experiences of suffering, and I know I will think of you and yours and how you have coped with honesty, grace, and spirit, and it will help me.

Linda G < 6/7/2011 8:55 AM >

We knew He'd use this challenge of yours for a greater good... looks like this might be it!! Praise the Lord!

Amazing! Your situation has definitely resulted in a serious ripple effect. God is using all of this for good. And I do believe your recovery will be the best piece of it!! Love you.

Debbie M < 6/7/2011 9:00 AM >

Congratulations!! It's nice to know that something positive, long-lasting, and of great benefit to others came out of your experience. Good on ya.

Joelle C < 6/7/2011 9:03 AM >

You are amazing! Galvanizing all of us to action even in the midst of your suffering! Brava, dear Robin!

Barbara C < 6/7/2011 10:37 AM >

This is wonderful news Robin. Good on all of us. I think I'll nominate you for a prize next year! I'd love to come up and help with the gardening, but I've now sprouted Harry's cold so I am infectious and feeling lousy. Put me on the list for something later, ok?

Kym H < 6/7/2011 11:05 AM >

Robin!! This is such great news and it's all due to your fighting spirit! YOU, my friend, are to be congratulated. You have changed the face of cancer in Nova Scotia for patients with rectal cancer forever! You are amazing and inspire me to achieve personal goals no matter what the barriers!

See you Sunday.

Patricia B < 6/7/2011 7:03 PM >

I think it was YOU that made all the difference in the FOLFOX approval—you pointed the many people who love you in the right direction and got us fired up! I am happy for all the cancer patients in NS who will benefit from this leap forward.

The Victoria Hospital sounds like a nightmare. I sincerely hope that you never have to go back there again. Is there no access to private rooms?

Are you back on solid food now and eating anything you want? I think slow-going and rabbit pellets are preferable to uncontrolled diarrhea—and easier to plan for on outings. Wish I could help with your gardening chores. Enjoy the nice weather.

Heather H < 6/8/2011 10:38 AM >

Well done to you, Robin. You've had many more battles than you probably would have expected and you have met them all with grace, humour, and determination. I look forward to reading your book!

I decide to congratulate the politicians involved:

From: Robin McGee
To: Tracey Preeper, Jim Morton, Kathryn Morse, Stephen McNeil, Maureen MacDonald, Diana Whalen
Sent: Monday, 13 June, 2011 11:42 PM
Subject: FOLFOX recommended for stage III rectal cancer

Hello to you all:

You may recall me. My community and I lobbied for FOLFOX chemotherapy to become available to Nova Scotians with stage III rectal cancer this past year.

I am delighted to see that the Cancer Systemic Therapy Policy Committee voted to recommend the treatment in March 2011. The link below describes their recommendation. I further understand that the Health Ministry approved this recommendation in the past few weeks: http://www.gov.ns.ca/health/cancer_drugs/Oxaliplatin_Eloxatin/Record_Recommendation_Use_Adjuvant_Rectal_Cancer. pdf.

Although this approval came too late for me to receive this treatment, I understand from my oncologist that several patients will start FOLFOX this week.

I want to thank each of you for your role in bringing this issue to the spotlight. You have all collectively improved the face of cancer care in Nova Scotia. This experience was an example of how an educated citizenry, in tandem with an enlightened government and a thoughtful Opposition, can work together to improve outcomes and save Nova Scotian lives.

Bravo to all of you!

Of all to whom I send it, only Diana Whalen replies, gently and thoughtfully:

From: Diana C Whalen
To: Robin McGee
Sent: Monday, 13 June, 2011 4:29 PM
Subject: Re: FOLFOX recommended for stage III rectal cancer

Dear Robin,

I am so glad to see that FOLFOX has been recommended for use and that some patients are beginning to receive it as a treatment for rectal cancer.

I very much remember your request that this drug be covered in NS and our inquiries to the Minister and the Committee that had to review it. I also heard from others who wrote on your behalf and it is clear that you have wonderful friends and colleagues who care greatly.

In closing, I just want you to know that hearing from you and your friends influenced me greatly and I so admire you for all you have done. Words seem so inadequate, but I wanted to reply to your email so that you know that when Tracey and I learned of the availability of this treatment in Ontario and not here, we were very concerned. The speed at which committees and government work is so slow. Thank you for writing to tell us of the change in policy and keeping us informed.

Thinking of you,

Diana

As a one-time student of English literature, I know that in the end, it all comes down to character. After all, it is what we have done that makes us what we are. It is my belief that Doctors One through Four each neglected me because of flaws within their characters. In my opinion, Dr. One had been ignorant, Dr. Two had been dismissive, Dr. Three had been lazy, and Dr. Four had been false. With differing motives, each one approached my case superficially because that was the easy way out of responsibility. But my salvation, and that of other Nova Scotians, hinged on the characters of those who do and did the right thing for patients.

I could see that it was in Dr. McIntyre's *character* to be professional and meticulous. His competence emanated from within him, from *who he was*. Like a gruff fire marshal who grinds out the cigar on the pavement before he rescues the family from the burning building, his focus and dedication were simply natural to him. In that way, his heroism was of the highest kind: the professional who does not know he is a hero, because he practices with excellence every day as a matter of course.

Character lay at the heart of the FOLFOX triumph. Judy McPhee did not have to call Dr. Dorreen—the Minister had already decided not to issue an exception in my case. But she chose to because it was her character to follow through.

I had been right to gamble on Dr. Mark Dorreen's character. A lesser doctor and a lesser man, called by the government on a case like mine, might have prevaricated. But he stood by his patient in a critical moment: when asked by McPhee if he supported FOLFOX in my case, his answer proved to be the pivotal moment in the story, without which nothing wonderful would have happened. His integrity in that instant, and his assiduous efforts to bring about best care for patients like me through the various committees, revealed his own quiet heroism.

And then there are the characters of others: of my MLA Jim Morton for bringing the matter forward to the Minister. Of Minister MacDonald herself, who authorized immediate funding for FOLFOX in the wake of expert opinion, despite fiscal pressures. Of Diana Whalen, whose compassion, diplomacy, and doggedness kept the issue on the forefront on the political agenda. And of each member of RCO who wrote to the politicians. Each one had thoughtfully composed a missive. Each one was a person of character: someone who cared for the stricken, believed in democracy, and who spoke out.

Finally, my story revealed to me my own character. The Robin's Cancer Olympics community was like burnished gold in whose reflection I could finally see myself. The community enabled me to be of good courage, and to plumb the depths of resolution required to live and to fight. I learned that a lifetime of character can be rewarded by a loyal and loving circle, and that good things can come about in a society of the just.

33

Recovery from the reversal is brutal. I have no rectum anymore. Reconnected without it, the missing body part is like a phantom limb. My mind sends familiar instructions to it, but nothing responds. It feels like waving an amputated hand in the air.

The frequency of bowel movements is unendurable.

OUCH OUCH OUCH
posted by Robin McGee, Thursday, June 9, 2011, 8:00 PM

Hello All:

This recovery process is much harder than I thought. Other colorectal cancer survivors had warned me: this part will hurt. And the continuous nature of the dysfunction and pain really takes it out of me. Yesterday, I lost count after over 20 trips to the bathroom. Today my skin is raw and bleeding. All the creams and lotions and baths do not do much to soothe, as they are challenged often within 10 minutes of application by more painful poops. My surgeon said this phase can last up to six months. It will take at least two years before my function will resemble that of a normal person, although I am told that I can never be normal.

Everyone treasure your functioning bum!

Sitz baths, lotions, baby products. Hours spent in pain. Dr. McIntyre declares my recovery to be unusually complex. Andrew quips that whereas our Queen had her Annus Horribilis, I was having an "anus horribilis."

I dread the thought of Dr. McIntyre's retirement. Who will look after me when he is gone? The enterostomal therapy nurses will no longer see me, since I do not have a stoma anymore. Nevertheless, ET nurse Eleanore Howard still keeps in contact, directing me to the best skin care. And Joan Hamilton, one of our "sexy nurses," follows up by phone and email. She continues to send me advice, remedies, journal articles, and encouragement.

....

The day of my final appointment with Dr. McIntyre is coming up. It will take place only days before his retirement after 25 years of surgery and 31 years of medicine.

I assemble the nomination package I had sent for the CCNS Excellence in Patient Care Award. I have my nomination cover letter, in which I extolled his history. I have the letter from a fellow patient. I have a letter signed by three enterostomal therapy nurses from across the province. But it is not enough. I decide to add a personal letter to him.

As I write, I am dizzied by the magnitude of the heights and depths of medical care I have experienced; but as the words form, I can feel myself healing. The emotion of gratitude spreads through my soul like a salutary balm. I smile as I realize that this is yet another way that Dr. McIntyre has rehabilitated me—he has given me a reason for respect. He has repaired my faith in medical care. Yes, doctors neglected me—but doctors saved me, too.

Wiping away tears, I write:

Dear Dr. McIntyre:

I get the impression that you are not one of those doctors who like patients to gush with gratitude. However, I want to take the occasion of your retirement to express my heartfelt thanks for all you have done, both for me and for all your patients.

By now you know it was me who nominated you for the CCNS Excellence in Patient Care Award. I thought you would like to see the letters I wrote and collected for your nomination. But these do not begin to convey the respect with which you are regarded by your colleagues. As my nomination letter states, so many of your colleagues identified you as not only the best colorectal cancer surgeon in the Maritimes, but the *best surgeon,* period. (Doctors Jean Gray, Daniel Rayson and Rebecca Dent were among those saying so). My Enterostomal Therapy Nurse Eleanore Howard said, "I can tell right away when I see Bernie McIntyre's work—his stomas are perfect. *Perfect.*" Dr. Mark Dorreen said, "I am so sorry to see him go...of all the surgeons, I trust him the most." When she heard I was seeing you, one of the oncology nurses spontaneously exclaimed, "Dr. McIntyre! That man is so gifted, I would let him operate on my child's brain tomorrow!" And Dr. Gillian Graves said simply: "He is a good, good man." At the time of my recent surgery, I told one of the OR prep nurses that I had nominated you for the award. "If that nomination had been a petition," she said, "hundreds of us would have signed it."

I credit you with saving my life three times over. The first occasion was the day I first saw you. You and you alone knew what to do for me. When every other doctor was saying emergency colostomy, you gave me concrete advice on how to save myself. I followed your advice to the letter and was able to start chemoradiation safely. The second occasion was of course the cancer surgery itself. It was enough to restore my faith in medicine—no mean feat, considering the travesty of medical care I received before I met you. There are no words strong enough to convey my gratitude for that day. The third occasion was when you called me at home to reassure me about the iliac node involvement. Your words relieved me from the choking despair of believing I only had a 4% survival chance. If someone had told me two years ago that I only had a 50% chance to live the next five years, I would have been devastated. But when I heard it from you that day, I received that news with joy and hope. That moment gave me my first glimpse of the possibility that I might be cured. From that moment until the present, I have recovered psychologically, and the difference in my emotional quality of life cannot be measured.

And what can one say about my most recent surgery? After two gruelling and complex surgeries, you still took me on. Even under what must have been exhausting conditions for you, you still took the time (indeed extra time) to do a meticulous and thorough job. I am sure that kind of focused dedication is second nature to you. But to the rest of us, such rare integrity is a reason for marvel, for honour.

In my clinical psychology practice, I have saved lives by talking people out of suicide or by helping anorexics recover. But I cannot imagine how it must feel to have saved thousands of people over the course of a career. Literally physically saving them. I imagine thousands of grateful people blessing your name, as I do.

You and I both know that cancer may claim my life in the next few years. Even so, your intervention has given me the chance to see my only child graduate from high school in 2013. This means so much to me, and to him. But who knows? Maybe I will live till I am 85. If so, I will raise a glass to you every 14th of September for the rest of my days. And when I do, I will say of you the highest praise and compliment I can imagine, for I will say this: you are Bernie McIntyre.

May your retirement bring you all the rest and adventure you so richly deserve.

I put the letters into an envelope along with a retirement card, and I wait.

AN END AND A BEGINNING

posted by Robin McGee, Friday, June 24, 2011, 1:15 PM

So many endings right now.

Yesterday I saw my surgeon for the last time. He says I seem to be healing and that my function will just have to take time. He said that my surgery would have removed all nerves to the area, and that these nerves will need six months to a year to grow back.

Once our consult was over, I told him I had something for him. I reached into my purse and pulled out a thick package.

"By now," I said, "you have learned that it was me who nominated you for the CCNS Excellence in Patient Care Award." He was surprised and staggered—he had not known. I told him that in the package was a personal letter from me, as well as the entire nomination package—my nomination letter, replete with salutary comments I had collected from other doctors, a letter from another grateful patient, and a letter from three ET nurses. He was delighted, as was the audience of nurses and medical students who watched us. He was also greatly surprised to realize that I had been in cahoots on this award with his secretary for months. She and I had agreed between us that she would keep it a secret until after my second surgery, but it seems she never told him. I think she knew I was going to give him the package, and she wanted me to have the honour.

When he shook my hand to say goodbye, he shook it in both of his capable hands.

Joelle C < 6/25/2011 12:30 AM >

Dear Robin,

You never stop amazing me with your strength and fortitude. I am in awe of your determination. How pleased your surgeon must have been to have your nomination at the end of his career. This shows you have the grace to reward excellence and the integrity to punish mediocrity.

Marilyn C < 6/24/2011 2:43 PM >

Oh, dear, Robin. Your story of the surgeon brought tears to my eyes.

....

Home from my last visit with Dr. McIntyre, I step out into the June splendor of my back deck. The weigela is thick on the vines and the honeysuckle is budding. It has been one year—almost to the day—since my treatments began.

Wandering to my garden fence, I marvel at the peony blossoms nodding on it. I see something amidst the greenery. I reach among the leaves to investigate.

It is the Buddhist prayer flags my sister gave me, now tattered and spent. Moving to untangle them, I find nascent flowering vines have grown around them and between them, like a green and verdant promise. I cry aloud with surprise and delight.

What is it that evokes our reactions to the synchronicity of the universe to our grief and hope? Do they arise from nature herself, brushing beauty over the fragility of our lives like paint on an artist's canvas? Or do they surface in the stirrings of our own hearts, broken open by life and death to awaken to the great mystery behind all things?

34

CHRISTMAS IS COMING.

Recovery has been a marathon. I have learned that I have a condition shared by many patients after extensive rectal cancer surgery: low anterior resection syndrome. The condition I am left with is characterized by disorganization of elimination, resulting from the severing of the nerves during the resection surgery and damage from preoperative radiation. Undue frequency and clustering of bowel movements are the hallmark symptoms. I will take months, even years, to come to some semblance of normal function, as my nerves regrow and my brain adapts to my new internal architecture.

I reflect back upon the past six months. This past summer and fall has been a storm of joys and challenges. I shared with the RCO community at regular intervals as I very slowly regained strength and function.

FURTHER DOWN THE ROAD
posted by Robin McGee, Monday, July 11, 2011, 10:15 AM

Hello RCO:

No sooner do you post that you are doing better when a day comes along that burns you and rips you to pieces. Now things are settled again. *Sigh*. It seems that my recovery path will be much like that of other survivors, characterized by steps forward and other steps backward. I will have a zig-zag course, it seems. But what can a person expect who is missing a fundamental body part?

Yesterday, we went tubing on the Gaspereau River. For those who have never tried it, it is idyllically fun. A shallow river runs in a gentle incline. You recline inside a large tire inner tube and float downstream, whooping as you swirl over the occasional rapids. The entire ride is about one half-hour, moving under a green canopy with the sunlight coming through it. Life does not get better than that!

While tubing, I reflected how lucky I was to be able to enjoy it. It was the first time I have worn a bathing suit in a year. (I could not bring myself to swim while I had Flipper). Any act of body reclamation is a wonder to a cancer patient.

My scars are starting to whiten. I have now what I call a "Frankenbelly"—a large vertical scar with staple marks on either side, plus a small round scar where Flipper used to be. Given that they were cut through twice in 10 months, I will have a lot to do to get those abdominal muscles back into shape. I have contracted Sherry Swanberg, of Swanone Pilates and Training Studio, to be my personal trainer to help me to do just that once I am able (in about two months, according to the doctors). So I look funny. I suppose this means that I will never be able to launch that career as a porn star. Oh well...I guess I will just have to go back to being a psychologist.

Tomorrow is the one-year anniversary of my father-in-law's death. We will find some way to commemorate it. Maybe we will drive down to the ocean, which was Ron's true home.

Namaste!

SUMMERTIME

posted by Robin McGee, Monday, July 25, 2011, 10:30 AM

Hello All:

I continue to get better slowly and incrementally. Things are slightly more predictable—typically mornings and evenings—and definitely more comfortable. However, "things" are still very time-consuming and disruptive when I have my attacks. So much patience is still required.

I have been having some fun experiences. Last week, I visited Glenora Distillery in Cape Breton with three girlfriends. We listened to 70s music. We sang James Taylor's "You've Got a Friend" at the top of our voices. And this weekend we plan to see U2 in concert in Moncton, so I must bone up on my Bono.

I have had some tougher times as well. A few weeks ago, my doctor sent me a copy of the last consult letter he got from my surgeon. In the last line, Dr. McInytre had written: "Hopefully she will not recur but obviously her cancer was high risk and there is certainly a chance for recurrence." I must confess that I had spent the last two months focused on trying to normalize my bowel function, that I had taken my eye off my not-so-great prognosis. I was thrown for a couple of bleak days.

Kris Carr, who wrote *Crazy Sexy Cancer Tips* based on her experiences, says that one is allowed to wallow in sorrow over one's situation for three days maximum. After that, one has to just be brave and pony up and move forward until the event that triggers the next wallow. I try to tell mtyself that my remission may last days, weeks, months, years, or a lifetime. No matter how long it lasts, I do not want to spend those precious days in despair. So I move on. Spending time with friends really seems to help.

Yesterday I was reading a psychology paper on happiness. The writer specified four kinds of happiness which lead to "the good life": *Hedonic* happiness, based on sensory joys (e.g., eat, drink and be merry); *Prudential* happiness, based on feelings of satisfaction from enjoyed work or activities; *Eudemonic* happiness, based on living in a manner that actively expresses excellence of character or moral virtue; and *Chaironic* happiness, based on a sense of spiritual awe, gratitude, and oneness with nature or God. Positive psychologists are coming to realise that well-being is based more on meaning and virtue in life's tough-choice situations, and less on pure pleasure. One psychologist wrote: "the focus on the maximization of positive affect and the minimization of negative affect has led to a view of the happy person as a well-defended fortress, invulnerable to the vicissitudes of life...perhaps focusing so much on subjective well-being, we have missed the somewhat more ambivalent truth of the good life." To have wellbeing, we must reach out and touch the face of the trauma that challenges our joys, our meaning and purpose, and our connection to God and others. So that is what I must do, every day.

CRACKERJACK

posted by Robin McGee, Monday, September 19, 2011, 3:45 PM

Hello All:

I have just returned from the QEII, from a colonoscopy to check for recurrence. Praise God, there was no evidence of local recurrence.

Today I met my new surgeon Dr. Lara Williams. She seemed every inch the bright crackerjack that Dr. McIntyre told me she was. She was smart, perceptive, funny, straightforward, and knowledgeable. She was one of those wonderful specialists who walks in, shakes your hand, and says: "Hello I am Dr. Williams and I know all about you. I know you had X done on Y date, and that you have experienced Z symptoms since." It was such a tremendous relief to encounter someone who had CLEARLY read my file before meeting me.

Not only that, but she seemed right on top of what must happen next for me. My next step, in addition to having blood levels monitored, is to have more imaging to check for metastasis. I asked if we could consider a PET scan instead of a CT scan. (Each CT scan has the radiation of 600 X-rays, and I have had three in the past year). PET scans are far less radiation and are considered more precise for peritoneal cancer. She listened thoughtfully, agreed that there was a point to my concern, and said she would page my oncologist today to sort out this issue, and get back to me within a few days. Again, I was both pleased and agog.

I want to add that I have learned that the Colorectal Cancer Association of Canada has worked out a deal with a private Ontario clinic to do combined PET-CT scans on patients like me for half their usual price. If I cannot get a PET-CT scan here, I can fly to this Toronto clinic and pay $1500 to have one done. So I will do that rather than undergo another CT, if I must.

The Canadian Cancer Society runs a Peer Connection program, in which cancer survivors volunteer to provide telephone support to those undergoing treatment. I went in last week for the training. I met a man, a fellow volunteer, who underwent the same experiences I did—same cancer, same stage, even the same complications. Only this man has been blind since birth. It was very poignant and humbling to hear him tell of his experiences, of the loneliness and terror of fighting cancer without the aid of vision. For example, he described the mournfulness of the sound of his IV machine as he lay in his hospital bed, and the anxiety of not knowing what the sounds around him meant. Just when you think you have it bad, you meet someone like him who truly exemplifies courage and resilience.

And now the best part of recovering from a colonoscopy...finally getting to EAT!!

50 TOMORROW

posted by Robin McGee, Friday, September 30, 2011, 10:00 AM

Hello All:

Tomorrow is my 50th Birthday.

I hope to have a nice brunch with close friends tomorrow morning. If the weather holds, I may see some friends from the psychology association who will come to help plant daffodils. And I expect we will go to the Port Williams Pub for dinner. We might like to assemble our Beatles puzzle, listen to Beatles music, and play Beatles Trivial Pursuit. Andrew also turns 50 a few months from now. We have not settled on how we might celebrate our mutual birthdays under our complex circumstances.

I struggle with how to respond to this birthday. I am VERY GLAD to see the end of the year I turned 49, given its harrowing qualities. I reflect on how much stronger I am physically now than I was this time last year (which was just after my first surgery). I have been following the program of my personal trainer for one month now, so I am regaining my fitness. Some of the bike rides I have made throughout the glorious Valley on these crisp fall days have been as beautiful as prayer.

Alas, I have had to open my doors once again to Fear Robin in my Room full of Robins lately. My CEA levels, which measure cancer through blood, are rising. My levels are still within normal, but the doctors are concerned by the trajectory. This Monday, I must have the level taken again. If it is any higher, they want me to move to immediate imaging to check for recurrence. I have decided that I will go to Toronto to pay for the private PET-CT scan under those circumstances, given how much more sensitive that technology is. The private clinic says I can get in within the week. In Nova Scotia, patients cannot get PET-CTs unless authorized by a special committee. It is so ironic to me that I am the patient representative on the provincial standards committee, but I have to fly out of province to have timely access to a test that might save me. Very early detection is the only hope of those experiencing recurrence.

For a cancer patient, any indication of recurrence is a nightmare. I feel like a Jew of the Holocaust cringing in a basement, listening to the footsteps of the Gestapo on the floorboards above me. *Don't find me, don't find me*, I pray, trembling.

But I have nowhere to hide.

During my Yoga, I have been taught a pose in which you sit back on your heels and put your forehead on the floor ("Child's pose"). I like to think of it as worshipful, like the prostrations the Muslims do. When I do it, I try to mindfully surrender to the Great Mystery, and to summon strength from God for the next steps on my journey, whatever those might be.

CEA NEWS
posted by Robin McGee, Thursday, October 6, 2011, 9:00 AM

Hello All:

Well, things are always interesting.

A new development...

Suspicious that the rise in my CEA levels was confounded by changing the lab that measured them, my wonderful family doctor Adam Good and I agreed that I should have this most recent level taken at BOTH labs—that is, at QEII and at VRH, on the same day.

VRH gave me 2.34, but QEII came back at 1.4!! The two labs differ by almost one whole ML! This is a significant finding; according to the internet, the range of concern begins over 2.5.

Moreover, this seems to indicate that I am not having a genuine increase—rather, I am cruising within a range, but that each lab shows a different range. If you graph the results from the two hospital labs, you see two somewhat parallel lines.

Of course, more data is required to be certain of this hypothesis. However, it seems now that I can go from full throttle terror back to the usual level of terror.

I confess I broke out the Scotch last night and put my Beatles on full blast.

HALLELUJAH
posted by Robin McGee, Monday, December 5, 2011, 9:15 PM

Hello RCO:

Today I had some good news. My CEA level came down again for the second month in a row. Down to 1.4 from 1.89 last month—and this from the "high" lab. So I made it another month, and now I can move into December feeling relatively safer.

My son Austin sings in the Annapolis Valley Honour Choir. This year, they are singing selections from Handel's *Messiah*—including, of course, the famous "Hallelujah Chorus." Some of you will remember that I sent a link last year to a performance of the "Hallelujah Chorus" sung in a mall food court by its apparent patrons, and how astonishing that was.

This time last year, I went to the AVHC Christmas performance in a state of choking despair. I had recently learned that I was considered to have only a four percent chance of survival. I watched the choir with my blood freezing and my throat choked, thinking that I was experiencing my very last Christmas. I tried to drink in every vestige of beauty from the music. I tried to take solace from it. I tried to bend my mind around the unthinkable loss of leaving my family.

This past Sunday was the AVHC Christmas concert, one year later—and I am still alive to hear them. This time, I listened with rapture to their performance. When they sang the "Hallelujah Chorus," I wept again. But this time with joy.

Epilogue

As I come to the close of this book, I still do not know how it will end. In the two years since my treatments ended, I have had two PET-CT scans done in Toronto. Both have described me as "unremarkable"—never have I been so delighted to be described that way. But given the seriousness of my initial pathology, my prognosis remains guarded.

Rehabilitation was long and difficult. Physically, it took many tortuous months—in fact, an entire year—to regain bowel function to the point I could attempt full-time employment. Psychologically, I needed months of therapy to be able to move forward. Like many cancer survivors, I experienced painful symptoms similar to the posttraumatic stress disorder of combat veterans. Whenever I encountered a triggering stimulus, such as the smell inside a hospital, I would experience a full body shudder, and the saliva would come warm and plentiful to my mouth. With the help of EMDR-certified therapist Denise Perron, I was slowly able to integrate my crushing physical experiences into the broader narrative of my life. My flashbacks diminished and my reactivity was soothed. However, my fear of recurrence remains deep inside me like a stone sunk into a still pool. EMDR has allowed me to dwell with my desperate experiences in a mindful "now" in which I live daily: sadder, wiser, but accepting.

I returned to my full-time school board work in the spring of 2012, almost two years to the day of my diagnosis. Slowly but steadily, I have been able to regain my life as a working person and move out among schools again. In January 2013, I was able to re-initiate my private practice.

About a year after my treatments ended, I volunteered to become a peer mentor through the Canadian Cancer Society CancerConnections program. Since then, I have been matched over the phone with over a dozen newly-diagnosed people. Providing guidance, reassurance, and true understanding to those who are struggling, as I struggled, helps to give meaning to my past suffering. It dignifies my cancer experience and enriches my life as a survivor.

In April of 2013, the Canadian Cancer Society Nova Scotia Division made a video showcasing me as a CancerConnections volunteer.[3] Also, I joined the AVRSB's "On Board for Life" Relay for Life team and have raised over $5700 dollars for the Canadian Cancer Society over two years. The RCO community remains the major source of my fundraising.

In the fall of 2012, my mother was once again diagnosed with colorectal cancer. It was not a recurrence, but rather a new primary tumour. Like her first, it was right-sided. Although her CRC surgery went well, a follow-up PET-CT has heartbreakingly revealed the presence of two other primary tumours in her breast and esophagus. We are devastated.

In Ontario, where my mother lives, all CRC tumours are screened at pathology for evidence of a condition called "microsatellite instability (MSI)." This condition can sometimes be sporadic, but can also be the result of a genetic syndrome known as Lynch syndrome. My mother's CRC tumour tested as MSI-high. Because I had early-onset disease, being under 50 years old at diagnosis, our family pattern is strongly suggestive of Lynch syndrome. Currently, I await genetic testing.

I have learned that all of us are vulnerable to colorectal cancer due to the insults to our GI system that occur over a lifetime, such as infections or viruses. For most of us, it takes approximately six decades to accumulate the approximately ten insults that trigger

3   http://www.youtube.com/watch?v=4-BkK4TsN_k&feature=youtu.be

colorectal cancer. In those of us with a family history of CRC, it may only take five insults. In those of us with Lynch syndrome, it may only take one or two insults. My own status has yet to be determined; yet I wonder if the antibiotics I had been given—the Ciproflaxin/Noroxin combination—was the insult that started my own carcinogenic cascade.

Lynch carriers have a 50% chance of passing the defective genes on to the next generation. If I test positive for Lynch syndrome, the next step is for my son and my siblings to be tested. Lynch carriers must receive intensive surveillance, such as annual colonoscopy starting as early as age 20, because Lynch tumours grow much faster than typical colorectal cancers. So perhaps my experience will allow my child and my siblings, and possibly their children, to be safer.

I have become extremely involved in cancer patient advocacy. In the fall of 2011, Cancer Care Nova Scotia (CCNS) announced the formation of an Oversight Committee aimed at developing standards of cancer care for the entire province. They wanted patient representatives. I volunteered and was selected to sit on this new Oversight Committee.

By coincidence (and to my delight), the first cancer targeted for improvement was rectal cancer. CCNS formed a working group to design standards of care for the treatment of those already diagnosed. The working group was comprised of surgeons, radiologists, radiation oncologists, medical oncologists, other specialists, and myself as the only patient representative. I attended dozens of meetings, which I sat through with my heart pounding, aiming to ensure adequate representation of the issues confronting patients like me. With great satisfaction, I have witnessed the experts endorse FOLFOX for high-risk rectal cancer, and I have seen it incorporated in the document as a *standard of care*—not a guideline, not a suggestion—but a standard. As I write, these standards are out for external review.

But recently I experienced something even more significant, even more compelling, even more wonderful and miraculous. Recently, I shared this event with the RCO community:

LIFEBOATS

posted by Robin McGee, Friday, April 26, 2013, 9:15 PM

Hello RCO:

Today marks the one-year anniversary of my return to work. I have worked full-time for one full year since coming off disability. A landmark, another island I have swum to.

It is the anniversary of another important event as well. As you may remember, I was working as the patient representative on the working group commissioned by Cancer Care Nova Scotia (CCNS) to develop treatment standards for rectal cancer. Issues of detection, referral, and diagnosis were in our terms of reference. However, because these matters are typically relevant to family physicians, they appeared to fall off the agenda of the expert specialists.

One year ago, 23 April 2012, another patient representative and I met with the Medical Director of CCNS, Dr. Carman Giacomantonio. We asked him to make diagnosis, and support of family physicians, a priority.

He listened, intently and respectfully. Within the month, CCNS had commissioned another working group. The mandate? To develop standards of care for family physicians regarding the detection and referral of patients suspicious for colorectal cancer. My fellow survivor and I were invited to serve on it, along with a team of family doctors, GI specialists, surgeons, and radiologists. The intent was to develop clear directives regarding the kinds of symptoms that require urgent referral (to be scoped in four weeks) and semi-urgent referral (to be scoped in eight weeks). Because Ontario had already done something similar, we had a template to start from. But we did something wonderful, above and beyond what Ontario had done—we developed a standardized referral form. This form is a checklist of key symptoms and risk factors that a family doctor can use to take a clear history from a patient when they refer for endoscopy.

Almost one year to the day we met with him—just last week—Dr. Giacomantonio and the Chair of the Diagnosis Working Group (Family Physician Heather Johnson) presented the detection standards to an audience of over 200 family physicians. The response was overwhelming: the family doctors had been desperate for better support and for faster timelines for endoscopy for symptomatic patients. The Chair emailed me afterwards to tell me I would have been so pleased. I told her that the audience was spiritually full of patients—past, present, and future patients—all giving her a standing ovation with grateful tears in their eyes. And that I was one of them.

For me, it has been a healing experience to work with doctors of integrity and vision. It was a curious relief to see that some family doctors actually do care about cancer detection. The great privilege is this: that I have lived long enough to see—and participate in—a systemic response to the mediocrity that resulted in my horrible, avoidable outcome.

Some of you know that the few survivors from the *Titanic* testified afterwards at an inquiry about the disaster. Like me, those passengers had been jeopardized and traumatized by the failure of those responsible to perceive real danger. Knowing that we will now have standards of care for colorectal cancer detection is like being a survivor from the *Titanic*, hearing at last that the shipping industry will from now on have enough lifeboats.

I cannot change my past, but I can transcend it. And I will continue to be a patient advocate for as long a time as I am given.

The RCO community continues to support me. Each announcement, like the one above, brings warm and cheering responses. My friends on RCO are still the stars by which I navigate my way home.

One day, FOLFOX will be replaced with superior cancer therapies. Recent news stories abound with hints from research showing novel successes and inroads against cancer. So one day, the fight for the FOLFOX regimen for Nova Scotians will be "old news"—a story, swept up like detritus into the ever-evolving history of science and medicine.

So what will be the lasting impact of this struggle? There may be long-term benefit to those members of my RCO community who were helped and encouraged. Perhaps this story might inspire other patients to lobby for needed change. Perhaps this story will inspire good doctors to continue to strive towards excellence and integrity. Perhaps this story will serve as a cautionary tale that will spook not-so-good doctors into being more careful with symptomatic patients, resulting in better cancer detection.

But to me, the power of my story lies in the faces of those who will be saved. Each year in Nova Scotia, approximately 1000 people are diagnosed with colorectal cancer—three every day. Improved access to the best practice chemotherapy will save dozens. Improved standards for CRC diagnosis and detection will save hundreds, even thousands. For my part, I will remain committed to ensuring that my provincial government will support the new standards.

As I confront my uncertain future, I wonder about the faces of those who will be rescued. I imagine someone's wisecracking brother, their affable father, their athletic son. I imagine someone's beloved sister, daughter, mother. I imagine someone's cherished husband or wife. These are the unseen faces that will comfort me when I die, whenever that day comes.

The psychologist had it wrong. There are not only four types of happiness. There is one he left out: *Relational* happiness—the joy that arises out of comradeship, out of love. The elated ecstasy of falling in love, the swelling warmth of cradling your baby, the steadfast feeling of devoted friendship.

There is another type of relational happiness. My Cancer Olympic journey taught me about the love of *community*, that ineffable presence whispering over the ether, with a susurrus as comforting as the sea.

Gratitude

SOME NAMES DO NOT APPEAR IN THE NARRATIVE, BUT ARE people for whom I am no less grateful:

For Ray Wagner Q.C. of Wagners Law Firm, for shouldering the burden of my terrible medical story when I was too sick to carry it alone anymore, and for carrying it ever since;

For Nicki Dennis of Dennis Publishing Consulting, for her editorial insight and encouragement with this manuscript;

For Allen Hume, Lesley Hartman, Thea Burton, and Janine Morin for their supportive comments on early drafts;

For Alex MacAulay of Alex MacAulay Photographers, for donating his time to make the striking cover photography;

For Geoff Soch and all staff at FriesenPress, for their dedication and patience in bringing this book to birth;

For Heather Rice of the Canadian Cancer Society Nova Scotia Division, for her commitment and perseverance with launching this book;

For Paula Huntley, for her verve and moxie with book promotion;

For Archie MacEachern, for being my comrade-in-arms over the long journey of cancer survivor advocacy and representation;

For Larry Broadfield of Cancer Care Nova Scotia, for teaching me the intricacies of cancer drug funding in Nova Scotia, and for his personal example of candour and courage;

For Jill Petrella of Cancer Care Nova Scotia, for her tireless efforts at bringing about standards of care for people like me;

For singers Ardyth Robinson and Jennifer Wyatt of Ardyth and Jennifer, for sharing the sublime gift of their harps and voices;

For singer Hal Bruce, for a rocking time of celebration for all of us; and

For Andrew and Austin Hurst, my husband and son. For everything. For love. For always.

About the Author

DR. ROBIN MCGEE IS A REGISTERED CLINICAL PSYCHOLOGIST, mother, wife, educator and friend. Living in Port Williams, Nova Scotia, she has been a dedicated clinician in health and education settings for over 25 years. Her work has included teaching at the university level and publishing in professional journals in her own field of child psychology. Since entering remission, she has been very active in patient advocacy, serving as the patient representative on several provincial and national initiatives aimed at improving standards of cancer care. She is also a peer support mentor and fundraiser on behalf of the Canadian Cancer Society. *The Cancer Olympics* is her first—and hopefully her last—memoir of her cancer experiences.

Please visit us at www.thecancerolympics.com.